# Mainstreaming Disabled Children into Physical Education

## Wonderful Adapted Equipment Ideas To Help You Mainstream Your Disabled Children Into Physical Education

**Christine B. Stopka**

**and**

**C. Patrick Sullivan**

University of Florida
Gainesville, Florida

KENDALL/HUNT PUBLISHING COMPANY
2460 Kerper Boulevard P.O. Box 539 Dubuque, Iowa 52004-0539

This edition has been printed directly from camera-ready copy.



ISBN 0-8403-7585-9



Printed in the United States of America
10 9 8 7 6 5 4 3 2 1

# Dedication

This book is dedicated to teachers everywhere who have succeeded, with their hearts and minds, to continually make this world a better place for all people.

# Contents

# List of Illustrations

## Figures

## Tables

# Preface

The purpose of this book is to provide you, the educator, with wonderful, exciting, affordable, buildable, and yes, really *do–able* ideas for using adapted physical education equipment to help mainstream disabled students easily and effectively.

Part One of this book provides clear illustrations and "cook book" type recipes on the construction (or "ingredients") of each major piece of equipment. Exactly how to build each device and where to buy the materials for approximately what price will be discussed. Furthermore, specific mainstreaming ideas and adaptations for each device's use will be included. Types of special populations who could use this equipment will be mentioned. National (AAHPERD: American Alliance of Health, Physical Education, Recreation and Dance) and state (DOE: Department of Education, State of Florida) physical education objectives will be identified for each piece of equipment as its use addresses and promotes the development of each objective.

Part Two of this book presents whole categories of equipment, discussed together such as, plastic bottles, ropes, boards, balls, etc., as well as the mention of any miscellaneous equipment ideas. These equipment categories and ideas are very inexpensive; indeed, most items presented can be home – made.

We hope you find this book to be useful. The illustrations have been made purposely as large and as clear as possible. *Please feel free to copy the ideas. The major goal of this book is to get this information disseminated so that all teachers can have access to these wonderful and simple ideas which should help mainstreaming become a rewarding strategy, rather than a fearful chore.* Hopefully, learning potentials will be maximized and a whole lot of fun will be had! Feel free to contact us if we can be of any further assistance to you or your program. Have a great time!

Christine Stopka, Ph.D., A.T.,C.
Associate Professor
Special Physical Education and Athletic Training
University of Florida
305 Florida Gym
Gainesville, FL 32611

Patrick Sullivan, M.S.
Retired, US Navy Pilot
Former PE Coordinator East Lansing School District
Present patient and volunteer
UF Special PE Laboratory
University of Florida
Gainesville, FL 32611

# Acknowledgements

The authors would like to thank the Department of Exercise and Sport Sciences, of the College of Health and Human Performance, of the University of Florida for their invaluable support given to the Special Physical Education program. In addition, the authors are very grateful to all of the teachers and special students with whom they have worked in the past as these are the individuals who have provided the purpose for creating such a book. Finally, the authors wish to thank their families — Rick, for his invaluable photographic contributions; and Sara, Dave, Katie, and Stephie for their unwavering support which made this book possible.

# Introduction

Please feel free to copy, adapt from, or use in any way, the ideas you find in this book. The simple, replicable, and clever devices are described in terms of how they are built and how they are used. Successful mainstreaming ideas are presented. In addition, both national and state physical education objectives are identified as each piece of equipment best facilitates their development. For a complete understanding of these objectives, please refer to **Figure 1** and **Figure 2** which display these objectives in detail.

**Figure 1** presents the American Alliance of Health, Physical Education, Recreation, and Dance's (AAHPERD's) five developmental objectives of physical education. Any program addressing these five areas of organic, neuromuscular, interpretive, social and emotional development is definitely on the road to quality, success, and accountability. References to these five objectives will be made within each discussion of the adapted physical education equipment in this book.

**Figure 2** presents the State of Florida, Department of Education's (DOE's) Curriculum Objectives for Physical Education (COPE). As with the AAHPERD objectives above, each discussion of the adapted physical education equipment will refer to these curriculum, or COPE, objectives, as the device facilitates their development.

This book will help educators identify appropriate objectives and content areas which will be enhanced by the use of each piece of equipment. The wonderful equipment ideas should help educators cope with the increasingly challenging task of mainstreaming a diverse group of students into already diverse and over–crowded classes.

# DEVELOPMENTAL OBJECTIVES OF PHYSICAL EDUCATION

## ORGANIC

Proper functioning of the body systems so that the individual may adequately meet the demands placed upon him by his environment. A foundation for skill development.

Muscle Strength
- The maximum amount of force exerted by a muscle or muscle group.

Muscle Endurance
- The ability of a muscle or muscle group to sustain effort for a prolonged period of time.

Cardiovascular Endurance
- The capacity of an individual to persist in strenuous activity for periods of some duration. This is dependent upon the combined efficiency of the blood vessels, heart and lungs.

Flexibility
- The range of motion in joints needed to produce efficient movement and minimize injury.

## NEUROMUSCULAR

A harmonious functioning of the nervous and muscular systems to produce desired movements.

Locomotor Skills
- Walking Skipping Sliding Leaping Pushing Running Galloping Hopping Rolling Pulling

Nonlocomotor Skills
- Swaying Twisting Shaking Stretching Bending Handling Stooping

Game Type Fundamental Skills
- Striking Catching Kicking Stopping Throwing Batting Starting Changing direction

Motor Factors
- Accuracy Rhythm Kinesthetic awareness Power Balance Reaction time Agility

Sports Skills
- Soccer Softball Volleyball Wrestling Track & Field Football Baseball Basketball Archery Speedball Hockey Fencing Golf Bowling Tennis

Recreational Skills
- Shuffleboard Croquet Deck tennis Hiking Table tennis Swimming Horseshoes Boating

## INTERPRETATIVE

The ability to explore, to discover, to understand, to acquire knowledge and to make value judgments.

A knowledge of game rules, safety measures and etiquette.

The use of strategies and techniques involved in organized activities.

A knowledge of how the body functions and its relationship to physical activity.

A development of appreciation for personal performance. The use of judgment related to distance, time, space, force, speed and direction in the use of activity implements, balls and self.

An understanding of growth and developmental factors affected by movement.

The ability to solve developmental problems through movement.

## SOCIAL

An adjustment to both self and others by an integration of the individual to society and his environment.

The ability to make judgements in a group situation.

Learning to communicate with others.

The ability to exchange and evaluate ideas within a group.

The development of the social phases of personality, attitudes and values in order to become a functioning member of society.

The development of a sense of belonging and acceptance by society.

The development of positive personality traits.

Learning constructive use of leisure time.

A development of attitude that reflects good moral character

## EMOTIONAL

A healthy response to physical activity through a fulfillment of basic needs.

The development of positive reactions in spectatorship and participation through either success or failure.

The release of tension through suitable physical activities.

An outlet of self expression and creativity.

An appreciation of the aesthetic experiences derived from correlated activities.

The ability to have fun.

**Figure 1:** **The five traditional objectives of physical education. This material is reprinted with permission from the JOPERD (Journal of Physical Education, Recreation & Dance), June, 1970, page 41. JOPERD is a publication of the American Alliance for Health, Physical Education, Recreation and Dance, 1900 Association Drive, Reston, VA 22091-1599.**

# PROJECT C.O.P.E.

CURRICULUM OBJECTIVES FOR PHYSICAL EDUCATION

CLUSTER I. THE BODY

A. SYSTEMS AND FUNCTIONS
B. CAPABILITIES AND LIMITATIONS
C. FITNESS COMPONENTS
D. EFFECTS OF ACTIVITY

CLUSTER II. PHYSICAL DEVELOPMENT AND CONDITIONING

A. AEROBICS
B. WEIGHT TRAINING
C. CIRCUIT TRAINING WITH EQUIPMENT
D. CIRCUIT TRAINING WITHOUT EQUIPMENT

CLUSTER III. LIFETIME SPORTS

A. ANGLING
B. ARCHERY
C. BADMINTON
D. BOWLING
E. FENCING
F. GOLF
G. TENNIS
H. PADDLE BALL

CLUSTER IV. TEAM GAMES

A. SOCCER
B. GATOR BALL/SPEEDBALL
C. MASS BALL GAMES
D. VOLLEYBALL

CLUSTER V. GYMNASTICS

A. STUNTS AND TUMBLING
B. FLOOR EXERCISE
C. VAULTING
D. BALANCE BEAM
E. UNEVENS
F. HIGH BAR
G. PARALLEL BARS

CLUSTER VI. TRACK AND FIELD

A. SPRINT AND RELAYS
B. DISTANCE RUNNING
C. HURDLES
D. JUMPING EVENTS
E. THROWING EVENTS

CLUSTER VII. MOVEMENT AND DANCE CONCEPTS

A. FUNDAMENTALS FOR MOVEMENT
B. CREATIVE DANCE
C. FOLK, SQUARE AND SOCIAL DANCE
D. SPECIAL RHYTHMIC ACTIVITIES

CLUSTER VIII. AQUATICS

A. DROWNPROOFING
B. SWIMMING
C. LIFE SAVING
D. AQUATIC ARTS

CLUSTER IX. RECREATIONAL SPORTS

A. RECREATIONAL GAMES — ACTIVE
B. RECREATIONAL GAMES — QUIET

CLUSTER X. COMBATIVES

A. SELF DEFENSE TECHNIQUES
B. WRESTLING

ALSO AVAILABLE:

INTRODUCTORY MANUAL

STATE OF THE ART SURVEY RESULTS

FIELD REVIEW REPORT

INFORMATION RELATIVE TO THE SECURING OF COPIES OF THESE MATERIALS MAY BE OBTAINED FROM THE PROGRAMS OF HEALTH AND HUMAN PERFORMANCE,
FLORIDA DEPARTMENT OF EDUCATION,
TALLAHASSEE, FLORIDA 32304

**Figure 2:** The Curriculum Objectives for Physical Education (Project COPE): the State of Florida, Department of Education, Tallahassee, FL, 1975

# PART ONE:

## A "Cookbook" for Adapted Equipment

## A. Archery Tripod

The archery tripod will provide an opportunity for severely physically disabled children to use a bow and arrow. This tripod will allow for these children to be integrated into an archery class, alongside their non–handicapped peers, with minimal assistance from the teacher.

1. Please refer to **Figure A–1** for a schematic diagram of this device. **Figure A–1** illustrates the steps needed for construction of the tripod from start to finish.

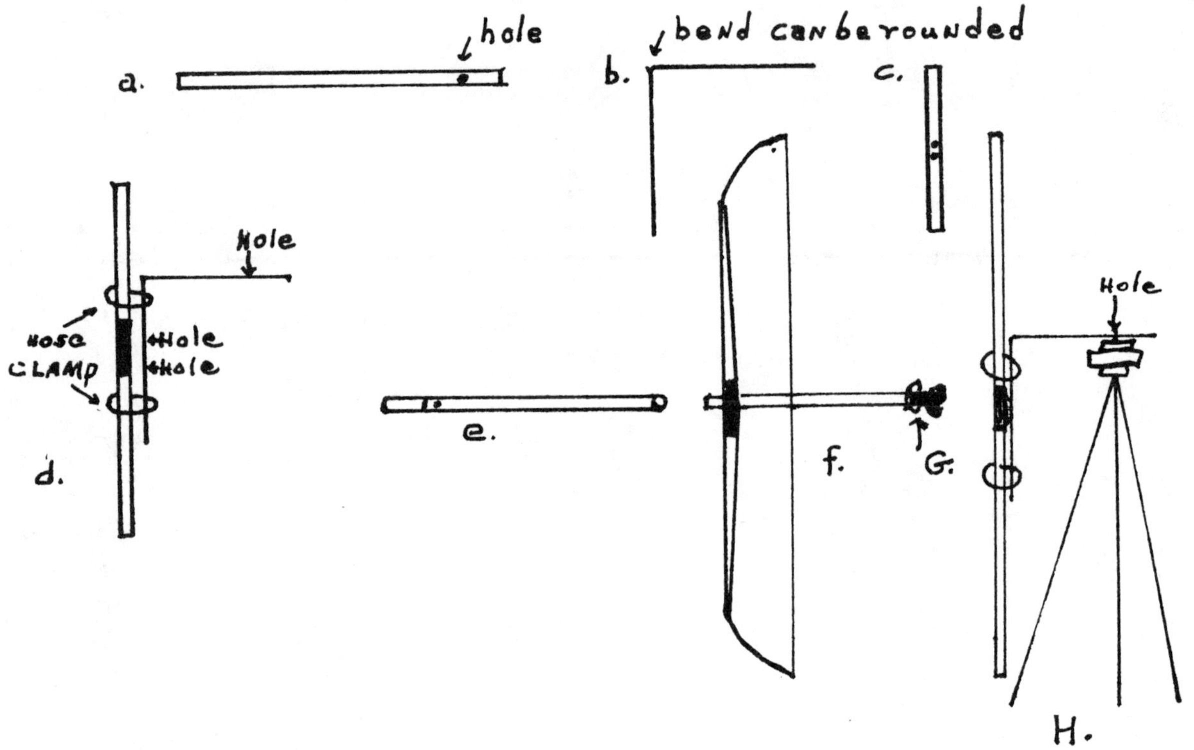


**Figure A–1**: Archery Tripod — Diagram

2. Please refer to **Figure A–2** (opposite) which are photographs of the actual device.

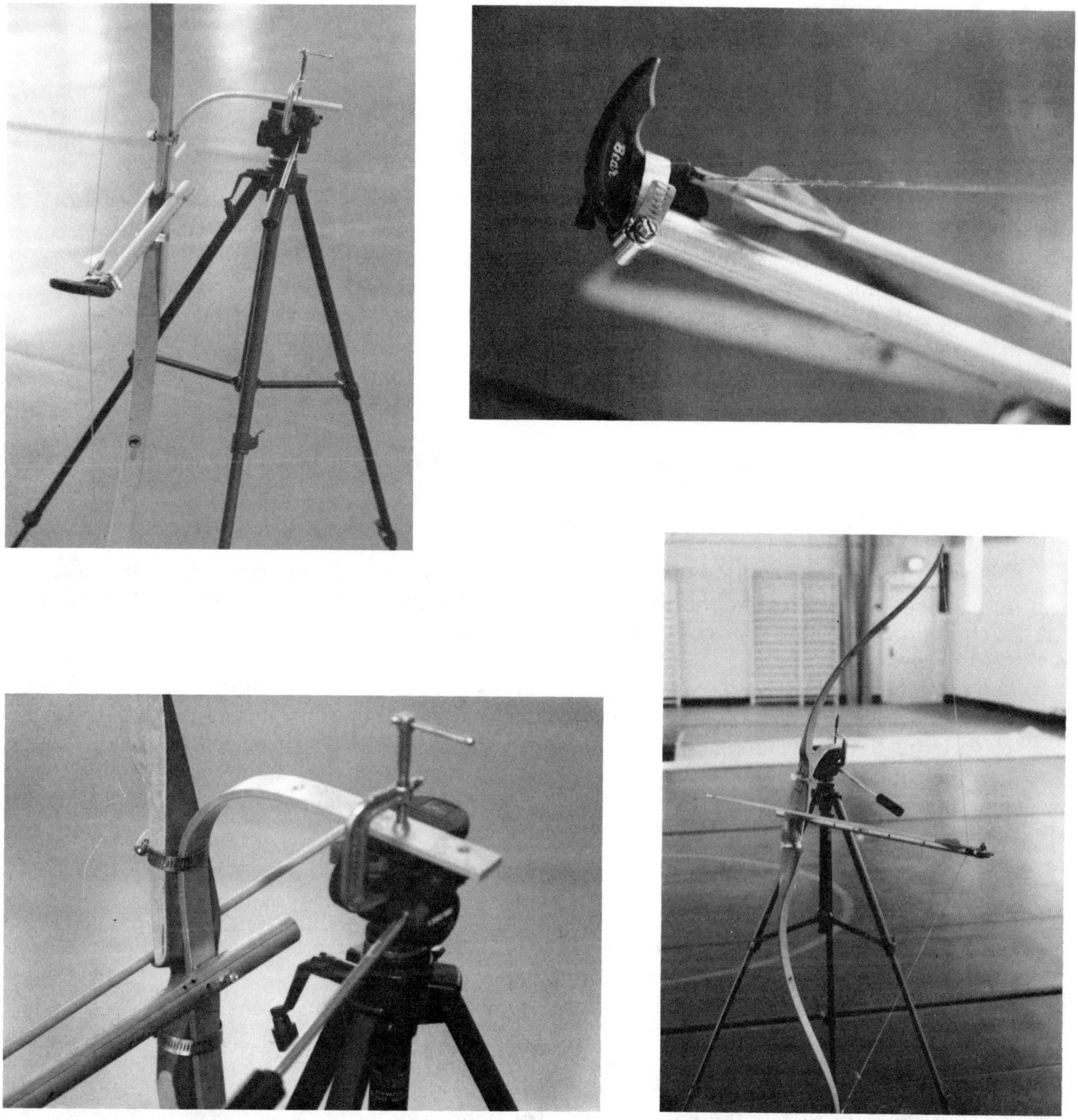

**Figure A–2**: Archery Tripod — Photograph

3. <u>What you need to build it</u>: The "ingredients" needed to construct this device are not hard to find. They consist of the following:

   a. One piece of strip aluminum two feet long, one inch wide and ¼ inch thick.
   b. One bow trigger (usually needs to be purchased at an archery supply store).
   c. One 3 inch "C" clamp.
   d. One bow.
   e. Three ½ inch hose clamps.
   f. One piece of aluminum tubing with a length three inches longer than the bow's pull.
   g. One camera tripod.

4. How you make it: The "recipe" or directions for constructing this device are as follows:

   a. Drill a ¼ inch hole three inches from the end of the aluminum strip.
   b. Bend the aluminum strip to a 90° angle (see **Figure A–1**).
   c. Drill two ⅛ inch holes through the strip at a spot which will match the grip of the bow.
   d. Attach the aluminum strip to the bow. Place the non–drilled end along the side of the bow and secure it with two hose clamps.
   e. In the aluminum tube, drill two ⅛ inch holes 3 inches from the end; these should match the holes drilled in the strap.
   f. Using ⅛ inch by 1½ inch bolts and nuts, attach the tube to the strip. The 3 inch portion of the tube should face forward.
   g. Attach the trigger to open the end of the tube using a hose clamp.
   h. Attach the top of the strip to the tripod using the "C" clamp to hold it firmly (see **Figure A–2**).
   i. Now you're ready to "fire away!"

5. How it works: The instructions for use are the simplest of all; just aim and fire! The firing mechanism works by simply pulling the trigger. All normal safety precautions necessary for any archery unit apply for the use of this device.

6. Other adaptations: Bows of differing sizes and tensions can be used according to the needs of the students. When very young children are using this for the first time, rubber (non–pointed suction tipped) arrows are recommended.

7. Mainstreaming ideas: The use of this device allows for easy mainstreaming. The children using this device can form their own small group alongside the other groups using the targets for the class. If the disabled child (or children) are severely involved, an able–bodied individual can help aim the tripod. The use of this device will provide an excellent opportunity for the educator to integrate disabled children into the class ***safely and very successfully.*** This device affords a high degree of accuracy; even the most severely disabled children can be known as the best archers in the class.

   a. Populations able to participate: All, even the most severely impaired.

   b. Examples of use: The easy to use trigger mechanism allows this piece of equipment to be successfully undertaken by even the most severely disabled. If the student's finger cannot be flexed to depress the trigger mechanism, a string can be tied to the trigger and student's mouth or even the wheelchair. The trigger is then pressed back by the student moving his/her neck in any direction or by moving the wheelchair backwards or sideways to tighten the string. Although an able bodied helper sets up the device, the disabled student can easily learn to give the positioning instructions in order to allow the arrow to reach the desired spot on the target.

8. Therapeutic benefits: Both national (developmental) and state (curricular) objectives are addressed with this device. Furthermore, therapeutic benefits involving the training of specific muscle groups can be facilitated with the use of this device.

   a. AAHPERD Objectives: This device addresses all five of the AAHPERD Developmental Objectives of Physical Education. See **Figure 1,** Introduction section of this book. Ranked in the conceivable order of their facilitation through this device are:

      1. Social: The device requires an aide for the most severely disabled, which necessitates social interaction. More importantly, whether or not an aide is needed, the device allows the handicapped student to be directly mainstreamed in a class of able bodied students.

2. Emotional: This device will enhance self–concept, etc., due to the feeling of accomplishment provided by the success of the experience.

3. Interpretive: This domain is enhanced as the student learns how to position, or tell the aide to position, the device for the best shot.

4. Neuromuscular: This domain is enhanced as it relates to the learning of fine–motor skills and recreational skills. Hand–eye coordination is practiced with this device. Fine motor coordination in order to grasp the trigger mechanism and pull it is addressed (or just pull it, without grasping, if the string adaptation is used).

5. Organic: Strength, endurance, and flexibility are minimally addressed when using this device with the most severely disabled. Less severely involved youngsters will have more functional control of their extremities and this domain would then be more developed. This should serve to convince the reader that even the most severely disabled students can successfully utilize this device.

b. State DOE Objectives: This device allows for the most severely disabled to conform to the State DOE (1975) curriculum objectives for physical education; Cluster III (Lifetime Sports); Section B (Archery). See **Figure 2**, Introduction section of this book.

c. Muscle groups trained: The wrist extensors (to provide a neutral position of the wrist against the use of the long flexor tendons) and the finger flexors, especially those supplying the trigger finger, are used. In addition the shoulder flexors and elbow flexors, to get the hand in position, are also used (unless the string adaptation is used, in which case the neck extensors and the chewing muscles (muscles of mastication) are used to activate the trigger). If the proximal end of the string is attached to the chair, the wrist and finger muscles used to operate the joy stick to move the chair sideways or backwards to tighten the string are used.

d. Other information: Whether or not this device is used, it is not always necessary to use official archery targets, especially in introductory sessions. A large "wall" of about ten or twelve bales of hay provides a great backdrop which is a large, safe target. This wall of straw for a target will help guarantee a successful experience for all children who can release the arrow in a forward direction. For further excitement and challenge, a rather densely packed array of balloons (or other targets) can be attached to the straw bales; if little space is left between the balloons, most all arrows reaching the wall will hit a target, thus providing wonderful, immediate, and very audible feedback for all to hear. As the children improve in the skill, use fewer (balloons) targets. Finally, visually impaired children will benefit greatly from the balloon targets (whether affixed to a straw wall or whether affixed to an official target) due to the immediate and obvious feedback they will get when their target is hit). The next section, "Archery for the Blind" specifically addresses adaptations for archery for those who are visually impaired (including those who are totally blind).

9. Notes:

## B. Archery for the Blind

"Archery for the Blind" will provide an opportunity for the most severely visually impaired children to use a bow and arrow. A sound device is placed behind the target to help the child aim the arrow. This idea will allow for these children to be integrated in an archery class, alongside their non–handicapped peers, with minimal assistance from the teacher.

1. Please refer to **Figure B–1** for a photograph of this adapted archery idea, taken just after a totally blind person shot his arrows (all of which successfully impacted the target).

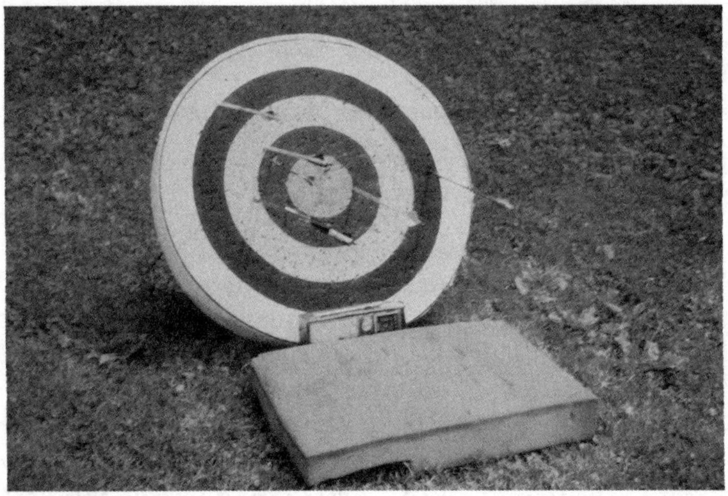

**Figure B–1**: Blind Archery — Photograph

2. What you need to "build" it: The "ingredients" needed to implement this idea are minimal. All that is needed is some sort of audible (and durable) *noise making device* such as an old radio, cassette player or beep ball — something that can be heard by an archer at the distance away from the target that is required for the event.

3. How you make it: The "recipe" is simple. A radio can be placed directly in front of or behind the target. If it is placed in front of the target, an added cushion or pillow is recommended to be placed in front of the radio in order to shield it from any errant arrows.

4. How it works: The student learns to aim and fire his/her arrow towards the sound. In a short time, the student archer will learn exactly how far above the sound he/she should aim in order to hit the target consistently.

5. Other adaptions: The use of balloons fastened to the target will help blind students gain immediate feedback regarding their aiming accuracy. This balloon idea is very rewarding to all because when the student's shot is successful the feedback is not only immediate, but it is very positive and exciting. The loud "pop" lets the blind archer and the whole class know that the "blind kid" was successful again.

6. Mainstreaming ideas: The children using this adapted archery idea can form their own small group alongside the other groups using the targets. The use of this idea allows the educator to once again, easily and effectively integrate a disabled child into the "regular" class.

a. Populations able to participate: Any degree of visually impairment.

b. Examples of use: "Blind" archery is carried out precisely the same way as archery for the sighted is done, except that a noise maker (such as an old radio) is used directly in front of, or behind, the target so that the blind archer can aim the arrows towards the sound.

7. Therapeutic benefits: Both national (developmental) and state (curricular) objectives are addressed by the use of this adapted archery idea. Therapeutic benefits involving the training of specific muscle groups can be facilitated by the employ of this technique.

a. AAHPERD Objectives: This technique addresses all five of the AAHPERD Developmental Objectives of Physical Education. See **Figure 1**, Introduction section of this book. Ranked in the conceivable order of their facilitation through this device are:

1. Neuromuscular: This domain is enhanced as the student learns a new sport skill. Ear–hand coordination is addressed and trained.

2. Emotional: This archery technique will help develop self–concept as the student gains in confidence with the knowledge that a new skill can be learned easily and successfully.

3. Social: This archery technique allows for the easy mainstreaming of blind and visually impaired children into a "regular" physical education class with minimal special assistance. The sighted students will learn and appreciate that even visually impaired children can participate and succeed alongside everyone and learn a new skill at a similar pace. The blind/VI children will begin to feel a greater sense of belonging and acceptance. Cooperation skills are enhanced as this idea allows for the children to help each other; it does not require constant teacher intervention.

4. Interpretive: This domain is enhanced as the blind/VI student learns to make his/her own decisions related to aiming adjustments, from the feedback provided by the sighted students (or the balloon adaptation, or feeling the arrows, or lack of them, on the target when retrieving the arrows, etc.).

5. Organic: Basic strength, endurance, and flexibility of the upper extremities and trunk are facilitated as the student works on drawing, aiming, and releasing the arrow successfully.

b. State DOE Objectives: This adapted archery technique allows the visually impaired to conform to the State of Florida, Department of Education, Curriculum Objectives for physical Education (1975), for Cluster III (Lifetime Sports); Section B (Archery). See **Figure 2**, Introduction section of this book.

c. Muscle Groups Trained: The bow hand's wrist extensors, elbow extensors, and shoulder flexors are utilized in this skill. The arrow hand's long finger flexors, finger intrinsics, elbow flexors, and shoulder extensors are also utilized in this skill. Back and trunk extensors help to stabilize the trunk and shoulder girdle for the desired upper extremity action. Anti–gravity muscles used for standing are trained somewhat (calves, anterior tibial muscles, quadriceps, gluteal muscles, hamstrings, and back extensors).

d. Other Information: See section A–8d in the previous "Archery Tripod" discussion for further helpful information.

8. Notes:

## C. Adapted Fishing Apparatus

The adapted fishing apparatus will provide an opportunity for severely physically disabled children to fish. This device will allow these children to enjoy fishing alongside their non–handicapped peers, with minimal assistance from others.

1. Please refer to **Figure C–1** for schematic diagrams, which illustrate the construction sequence of this device from start to finish.

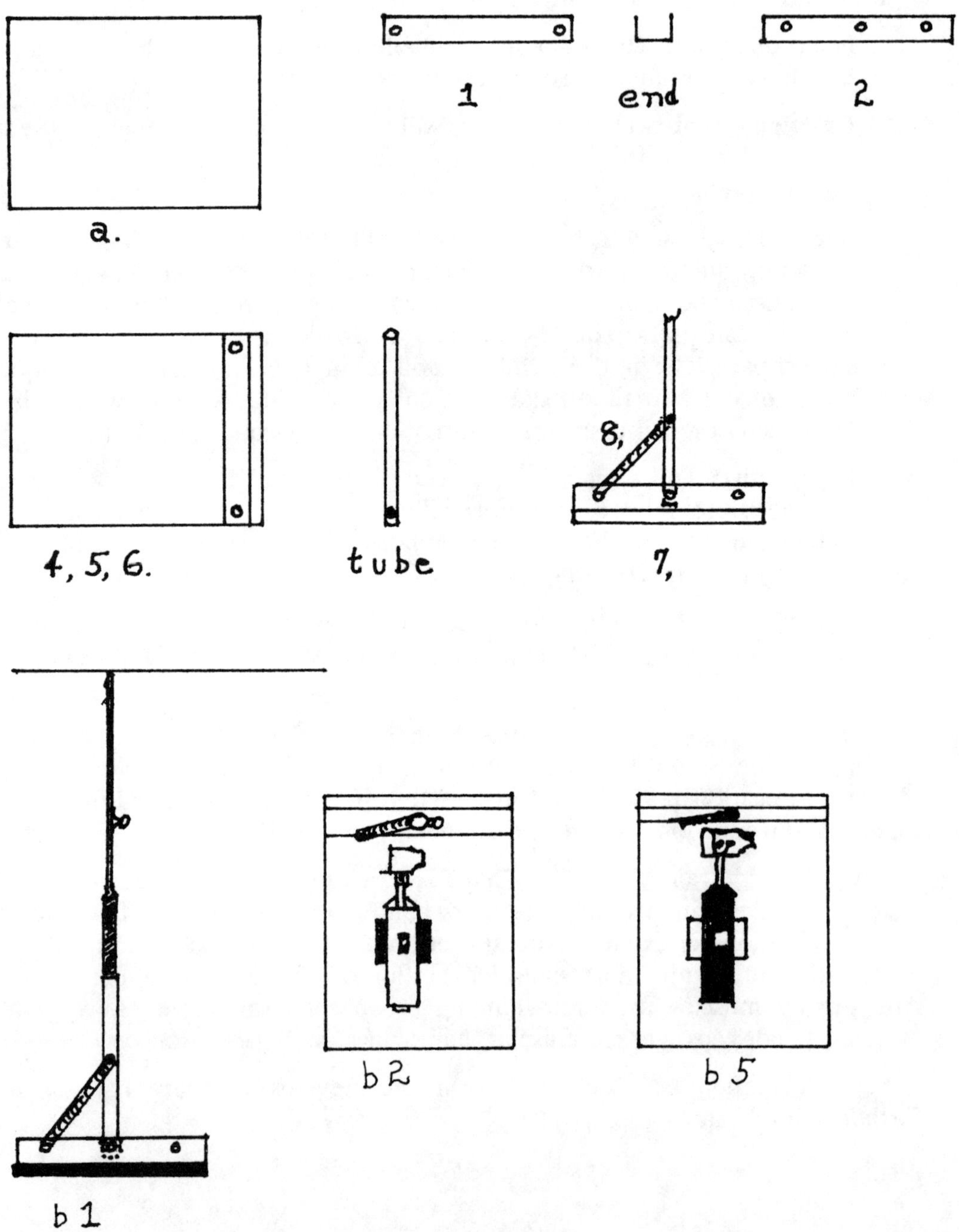


**Figure C–1**: Adapted Fishing Apparatus — Diagram

2. Please refer to **Figure C–2** which are photographs of the actual device.

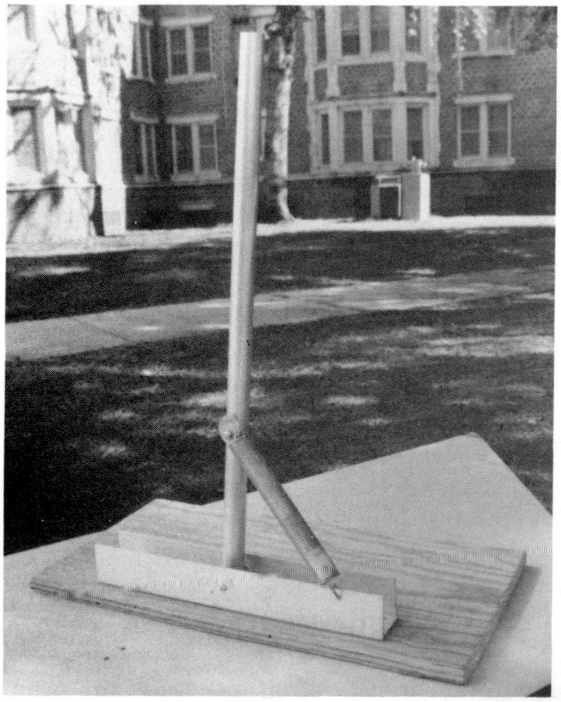

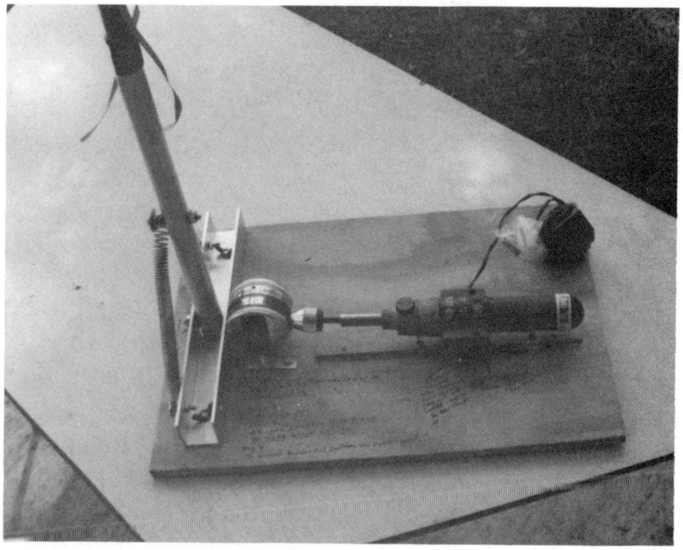

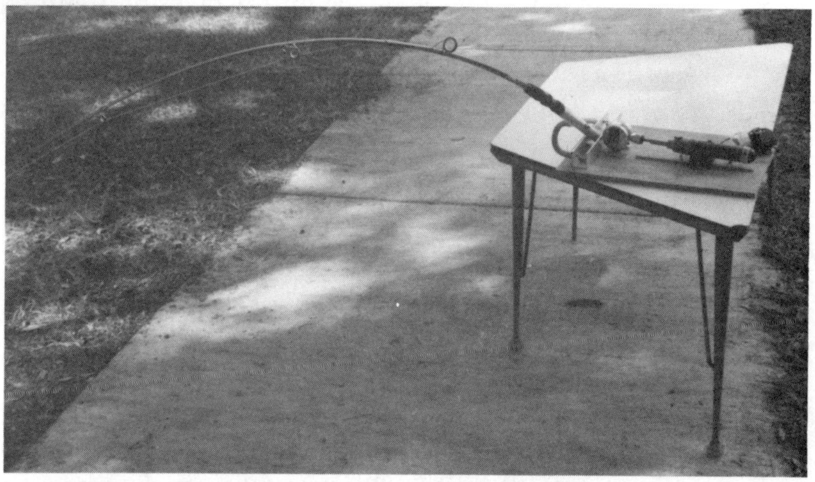

**Figure C–2**: Adapted Fishing Apparatus — Photograph

3. What you need to build it: The "ingredients" needed to construct this device are not hard to find. They consist of the following:

   a. One piece of aluminum tracking material 15 inches long and at least 1½ inches wide and 1½ inches deep (see **Figure C–2**).
   b. One piece of ¾ inch plywood at least 20 inches long and 16 inches wide.
   c. A coil spring (about ½ inch to 1 inch in diameter, depending on the amount of flinging power desired).
   d. One piece of aluminum tubing 1 inch in diameter by 15 inches long.

   Note: Items a–d constitute the "flinger power unit" which will also be utilized in other devices to be discussed shortly.

e. A spinning (fishing) rod and reel.
f. A battery powered screw driver.
g. A socket wrench.
h. Two wood screws, which generally come with the screw driver.

4. How you make it: The "recipe" or directions for building this device, including the flinger unit, are as follows:

   a. Flinger unit:

      1. Prepare the tracking; drill a ¼ inch hole 1 inch from each end of the bottom of the track.
      2. Drill *holes through both sides* of the track, locating the holes ½ inch from the top, one 2 inches from each end, and through the middle of the side.
      3. Mount the track on the board; align the track 1 inch from the 16 inch edge of the board.
      4. Mark the position of the holes in the bottom of the track and drill ¼ inch holes through the board.
      5. Attach the track to the board with ¼ inch and 1¼ inch nuts and bolts. The head of the bolt should be on the underside of the board.
      6. Attach the aluminum tube to the track. Drill a ¼ inch hole through either end of the tube. Place the drilled end of the tube in the track and secure by running a ¼ inch bolt through both sides of the track and tube.
      7. Attachment of the spring: Attach the spring using the hole at either end of the track. Holding the tube straight up, take the free end of the spring and mark point where it meets the tube.
      8. Drill a ¼ inch hole through the tube and attach the spring to the tube with ¼ inch by 1¼ inch bolt and nut.

   b. Rod and reel attachment to the flinger unit:

      1. Insert spinning rod handle into aluminum tube of the flinger power unit.
      2. Mount the reel on the plywood board base with the handle away from the power unit and the front of the reel even with the rod and the aluminum tube.
      3. Remove winding handle from the reel. Replace the nut which held the handle.
      4. Mount the screw driver on the charger and place the socket wrench in the screwdriver.
      5. Slide the socket wrench over the nut which held the handle.
      6. Press the charging unit against the base (the plywood board) and hold it firmly.
      7. Remove the screwdriver and mark the screw holes in the charger on the base board.
      8. Prepare the holes and mount the charger to the baseboard with screws.
      9. Replace the screwdriver socket wrench on the reel.

5. How it works: The use of this device is a relatively simple two step operation. The first step consists of casting the rod. The rod is cast by pulling the pole backwards, or cocking it, to tighten the tension of the spring. When the rod is cocked, the student merely lets it loose, i.e., lets go of the rod. This will cause the spring to let the end of the rod, and the bait, fly forward toward the water. (The device, fitted with an average size spring, allows for an easy 30 to 40 foot casting range). When the bait is set, the student can easily reel the "catch" in by depressing the "on" button on the "screw driver" attachment.

6. Other adaptations: The most severely disabled students may need help depressing the release button on the rod to allow the line to feed during the cast. Also, depending on how well the

device is bolted down, the student may need someone to steady the device due to the high amount of torque produced by the casting spring.

Students who are not quite so severely disabled, such as those having functional use of at least one arm and hand may opt to forego the casting spring and "screw driver reel in" features. They may wish to cast with the one hand, place the rod in a chest "holster" and then use the functional hand to wind the line to reel in the "catch." The stability of the pole is provided for by a chest holster, rather than the other hand.

Finally, students who have good use of one hand and only partial use of the other may wish to cast with the lesser functional hand with the help of the rod being secured to the hand and wrist with a bowling glove and reel the catch in with the more functional hand. Specifically, the ingredients needed to build this fishing rod for the less impaired are:

a. One casting rod and reel.
b. One bowling glove (get a good quality one with metal support built into the palm side and back side of the glove).
c. Two ⅛ inch by 2 inch bolts with nuts.

The procedure for constructing this rod is the following:

a. Place the palm of the bowling glove against the side of the rod handle and mark two spots where holes can be drilled through both the glove and the handle.
b. Remove the glove and drill the holes.
c. Replace the glove and mark holes on the handle of the casting rod.
d. Drill holes in the handle.
e. Attach the glove to the rod handle (from the glove side and through the rod) using ⅛ inch by 2 inch bolts (this places the nuts away from the hand).

7. Mainstreaming ideas: The children using these devices can "fish" alongside other students. The use of these adapted fishing ideas allows for the easy and effective integration of disabled children into a "regular" class.

   a. Populations able to participate: All, even the most severely impaired.

   b. Examples of use: The adapted fishing apparatus, along with its aforementioned variations, can be used in any lifetime sports unit teaching casting and fishing. *Also*, since the motion is somewhat similar to various throwing motions, these adapted fishing devices could be used for handicapped children during the instruction of other physical education/sports teaching units.

8. Therapeutic benefits: Both national (developmental) and state (curricular) objectives are addressed with the adapted fishing apparatus and its variations. Furthermore, therapeutic benefits involving the training of specific muscle groups can be facilitated with the use of these devices.

   a. AAHPERD Objectives: This device addresses all five of the AAHPERD Developmental Objectives of Physical Education. See **Figure 1**, Introduction section of this book. Ranked in the conceivable order of their facilitation through these devices are:

      1. Neuromuscular: This domain is enhanced as the student learns a new sport/lifetime recreational skill.

      2. Emotional: These "fishing" devices help develop self–concept as the student gains in confidence with the knowledge that a new and generalizable skill can be learned easily and successfully.

3. Social: These "fishing" devices allow for the easy mainstreaming of even the most severely disabled children into a "regular" physical education class. Cooperation skills are enhanced as children learn to assist each other with the devices.

4. Interpretive: This domain is enhanced as the child learns how to operate these devices well enough to "fish" successfully. Many cognitive concepts such as directionality, space, time, speed, force, safety, strategy, and others are addressed and experienced by children utilizing these devices.

5. Organic: Basic strength, endurance, and flexibility are minimally addressed when using these devices. The hand held adaptation for the lesser disabled will result in more training of these areas than the other, more passive devices presented.

b. State DOE Objectives: This device allows for even the most severely disabled children to conform to the State DOE (1975) curriculum objectives for physical education; Cluster IX (Recreational Sports); Section B (Quiet Recreational Games). See **Figure 2**, Introduction section of this book.

c. Muscle groups trained: The wrist and finger flexors are used, if the child is able, even with the most automatic, passive fishing adaptation, as the child cocks the pole back to engage the spring loaded casting mechanism. Elbow flexors help to pull the pole back, and shoulder extensors take over to keep the pole cocked until it is time to release it. Students able to use the more active, hand held devices, engage the shoulder and elbow flexors, as well as the wrist extensors during the cocking phase. During the casting phase, they utilize the shoulder extensors, elbow extensors, and wrist flexors.

9. Notes:

## D. Frisbee Flinger

The frisbee flinger will provide an opportunity for severely physically disabled children to throw a frisbee. This device will allow these children to participate in frisbee games alongside their non-handicapped peers, with minimal assistance from others.

1. Please refer to **Figure D–1** for schematic diagrams which illustrate the construction sequence of this device from start to finish.

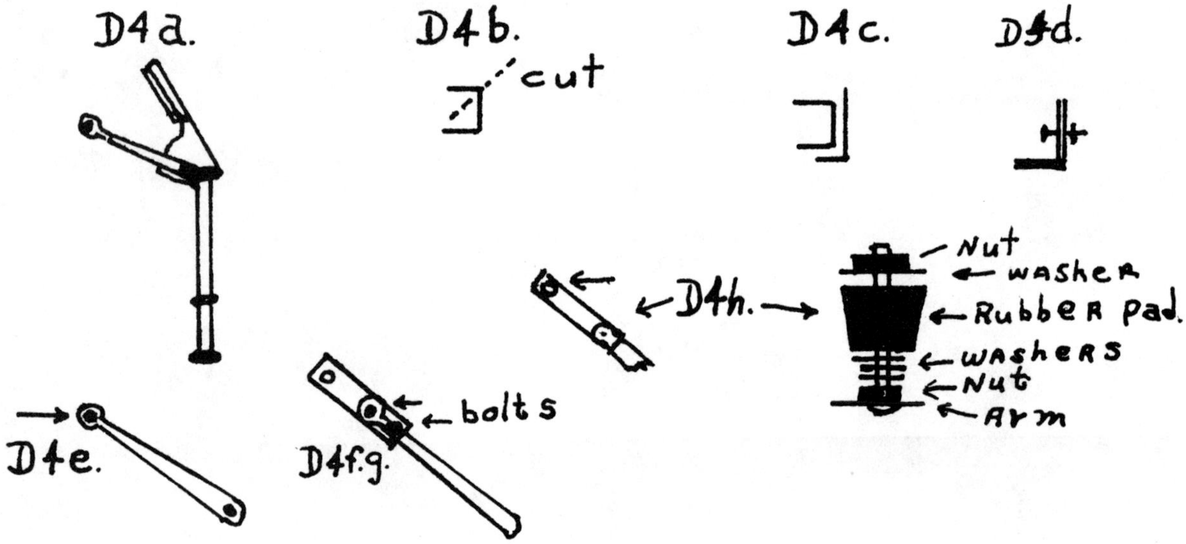


**Figure D–1**: Frisbee Flinger — Diagram

2. Please refer to **Figure D–2** which are photographs of the actual device.

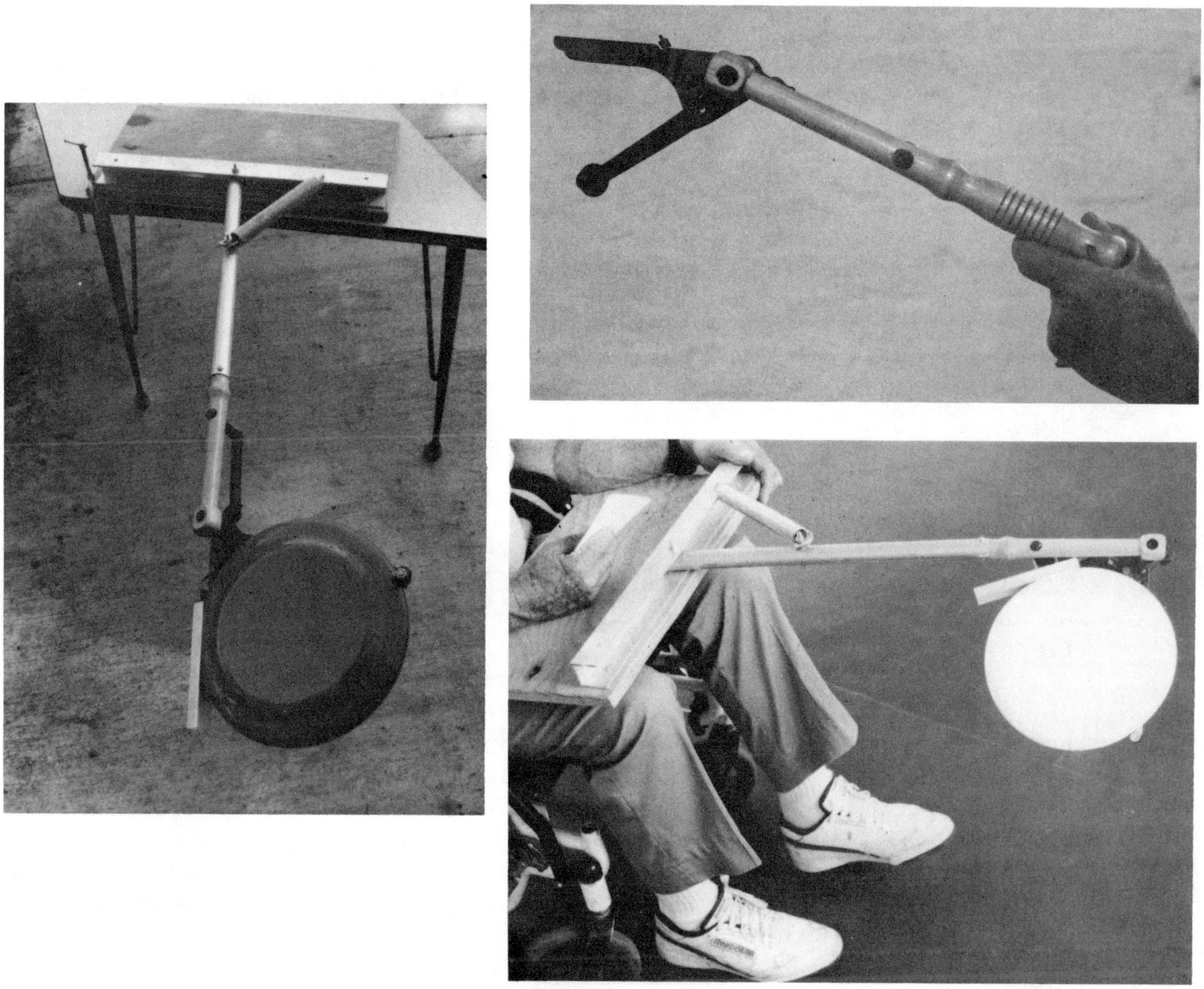

**Figure D–2**: Frisbee Flinger — Photograph

3. <u>What you need to build it</u>: The "ingredients" needed to construct this device are not hard to find. They consist of the following:

   a. One flinger unit (described in Section C, above: The Adapted Fishing Apparatus). This flinger unit should be placed on its side at the end of the board and bolted in place (see **Figure D–1a**).

   b. One hand held clay target thrower (can be found in the sporting goods department of stores like Wal–Mart and K–Mart).

   c. One 6 inch piece of aluminum window tracking material which measures $\frac{7}{8}$ of an inch wide and $\frac{1}{2}$ inches high.

   d. A metal strip 5 inches long, $\frac{3}{4}$ inches wide and 1/16 of an inch thick.

   e. Five nuts and bolts $\frac{3}{4}$ inches long and 3/16 inches in diameter.

   f. Four nuts and bolts $1\frac{1}{4}$ inches long and 3/16 inches in diameter.

4. How you make it: The "recipe" or directions for building this device are as follows:
   a. There are two arms on the target thrower: One arm is stationary, the other arm is attached to a spring and can be moved. It is necessary to lengthen each of these arms so that they will accommodate a frisbee.
   b. On the forward end of the fixed arm you will find a three sided channel. Cut off the top side of this channel leaving the end of the arm with the bottom and back intact (see **Figure D–1b**).
   c. Place the 6 inch piece of aluminum tracking on the arm so that the back edges of the two tracks are even and the open section faces the flexible arm (see **Figure D–1c**).
   d. When the track is in place mark and drill two 3/16 inch holes, 2 inches apart, through both back pieces. Push ¾ inch bolts first through the aluminum track and then through the stationary arm and attach the nuts (see **Figure D–1d**).
   e. On the end of the movable arm there is a rivet surrounded by a rubber pad; this rivet must be removed. The best way to remove it is to use either a file or a grinding wheel and remove the material on the bottom edge of the rivet (see **Figure D–1e**). Save the rubber pad.
   f. Place the 5 inch metal strip on the flexible arm so that 2½ inches extend beyond the rivet hole in the arm. Mark the strip and drill a hole to match the one in the arm (3/16 of an inch). Place the ¾ inch by 3/16 inch bolt through both holes and attach and tighten the nut (see **Figure D–1f**).
   g. About 1 inch toward the back of the strip, drill a 3/16 inch hole through both the strip and the thrower arm. Put the ¾ by 3/16 inch bolt through the hole and secure it with a nut (see **Figure D–1g**).
   h. About ½ inches from the front of the metal strip, drill a 3/16 inch hole. From the back side of the hole, push through a 1¼ inch bolt; place the nut on the bolt and tighten until the bolt is secure to the thrower arm. Next, add to the bolt three ½ inch washers, the rubber pad (narrow end first), another ½ inch washer and two nuts. Tighten nuts until all pieces are secure, but the rubber pad can still turn (see **Figure D–1h**).
   i. The frisbee thrower is now ready to be placed on the power unit (i.e., the flinger unit). The best way to do this is to reduce the size of the handle so that it will fit into the throwing arm of the power unit. This can be accomplished by using a knife, saw, wood chisel or a wood rasp.
   j. When the handle is ready to fit into the flinger arm, insert the handle, put the frisbee between the arms and turn the handle until the leading edge of the frisbee is approximately 30 degrees higher than the back edge. Drill a hole through the flinger arm and the handle of the thrower. Insert a 1¼ inch by 3/16 inch bolt through both the flinger arm and the handle and secure with its nut (see **Figure D–1j**).

5. How it works: The use of this device is a relatively simple, three step operation. The first step is to insert the frisbee into the adapted skeet shooter holders. The second step consists of cocking the skeet shooter section *and* cocking the flinger arm section. The third step is to merely "stand" clear and release the flinger (i.e., let go!). The frisbee is sure to fly a nice long, level distance of about 25 to 50 yards, depending on the size of the spring used and the wind conditions.

6. Other adaptations: The most severely disabled can operate this device at least partially. Some children may find difficulty in loading the frisbee and cocking the distal skeet shooter section. If this is the case, an able bodied assistant can perform this step, still allowing the handicapped child to cock the proximal flinger arm. The assistant can help stabilize the base of the device as the handicapped child releases the flinger arm. The frisbee will then take off perfectly, the assistant only having helped out with the initial loading process. Extremely disabled children can cock and "fire" the flinger by attaching a string to the flinger and their electric chair. When the

child backs up, the flinger is cocked. When the string is let go, the flinger fires, i.e., the frisbee flies off to its destination, aimed by the child.

7. Mainstreaming ideas: Children using this device can throw frisbees, play frisbee golf, essentially join in right alongside able bodied peers as they engage in any type of throwing unit. The device is portable and can be clamped to the wheelchair. The child can be integrated safely and effectively with his/her able bodied peers.

   a. Populations able to participate: All; the most severely impaired may need assistance with some of the cocking process; the flinging process is very simple.

   b. Examples of use: The use of this device would fit right in during any ultimate frisbee, frisbee golf, or other frisbee sport lesson. A disabled child could also be integrated into a track and field unit, as he/she could use this device alongside the discus or shot put events. This device could fit into any throwing, or target based unit; the disabled child would just be throwing frisbees, rather than other things (balls, whatever).

8. Therapeutic benefits: Both national (developmental) and state (curricular) objectives are addressed with the frisbee flinger. Furthermore, therapeutic benefits involving the training of specific muscle groups can be facilitated with the use of this device.

   a. AAHPERD Objectives: This device addresses all five of the AAHPERD Developmental Objectives of Physical Education. See **Figure 1**, Introduction section of this book. Ranked in the conceivable order of their facilitation through this device are:

      1. Neuromuscular: This domain is enhanced as the student learns a new sport/lifetime recreational skill.

      2. Emotional: This device will help build self–concept as the student gains in confidence with the knowledge that a new and exciting skill can be learned.

      3. Social: A sense of belonging and acceptance can be fostered as this device will allow the disabled child to join able bodied peers in frisbee games, such as frisbee golf, on an equal level of competition. Even the more severely disabled children can use this device with only minimal assistance from others, thus making it an excellent device to have to help integrate disabled children successfully in the program.

      4. Interpretive: This domain is enhanced as the child learns how to operate this device well enough to aim and fly the frisbee as desired. Many cognitive concepts such as directionality, space, time, speed, force, moment arms, levers, torque, resistance, lift, laminar flow, turbulence, strategy, safety, and others are addressed and experienced by children using this device.

      5. Organic: Basic strength, endurance, and flexibility are minimally addressed when using this device. The cocking phase of the flinger arm requires the most strength. Once the arm is cocked, engaging it takes little effort.

   b. State DOE Objectives: This device allows for even the most severely disabled children to conform to the State DOE (1975) curriculum objectives for physical education; Cluster IX (Recreational Sports); Section A or B (Active or Quiet Recreational Games). See **Figure 2**, Introduction section of this book.

   c. Muscle groups trained: During the cocking phase, the wrist and elbow flexors are engaged as the student grasps the flinger arm to pull it back to the cocking position. As the flinger is pushed and held down until it is cocked, the elbow extensors and forearm pronators come into play.

d. Other information: If the student is too severely disabled to perform the cocking phase independently, an able–bodied individual can assist with this phase partially, or even totally, as needed.

9. Notes:

## E. Racquet Ball Racquet

The racquet ball racquet will provide an opportunity for severely physically disabled children to experience hitting the different balls from a variety of racquet sports. This will help them acquire an appreciation for the demands of these sports.

1. Please refer to **Figure E–1** for schematic diagrams which illustrate the construction sequence of this racquet.

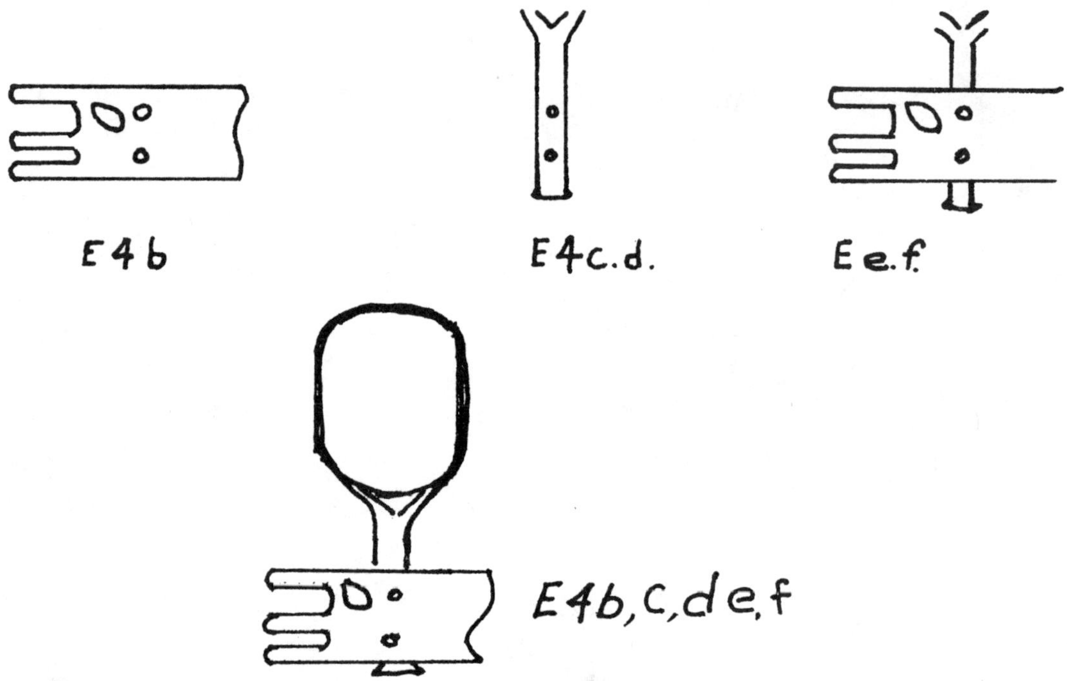


**Figure E–1**: Racquet Ball Racquet — Diagram

2. Please refer to **Figure E–2** which are photographs of the actual racquet.

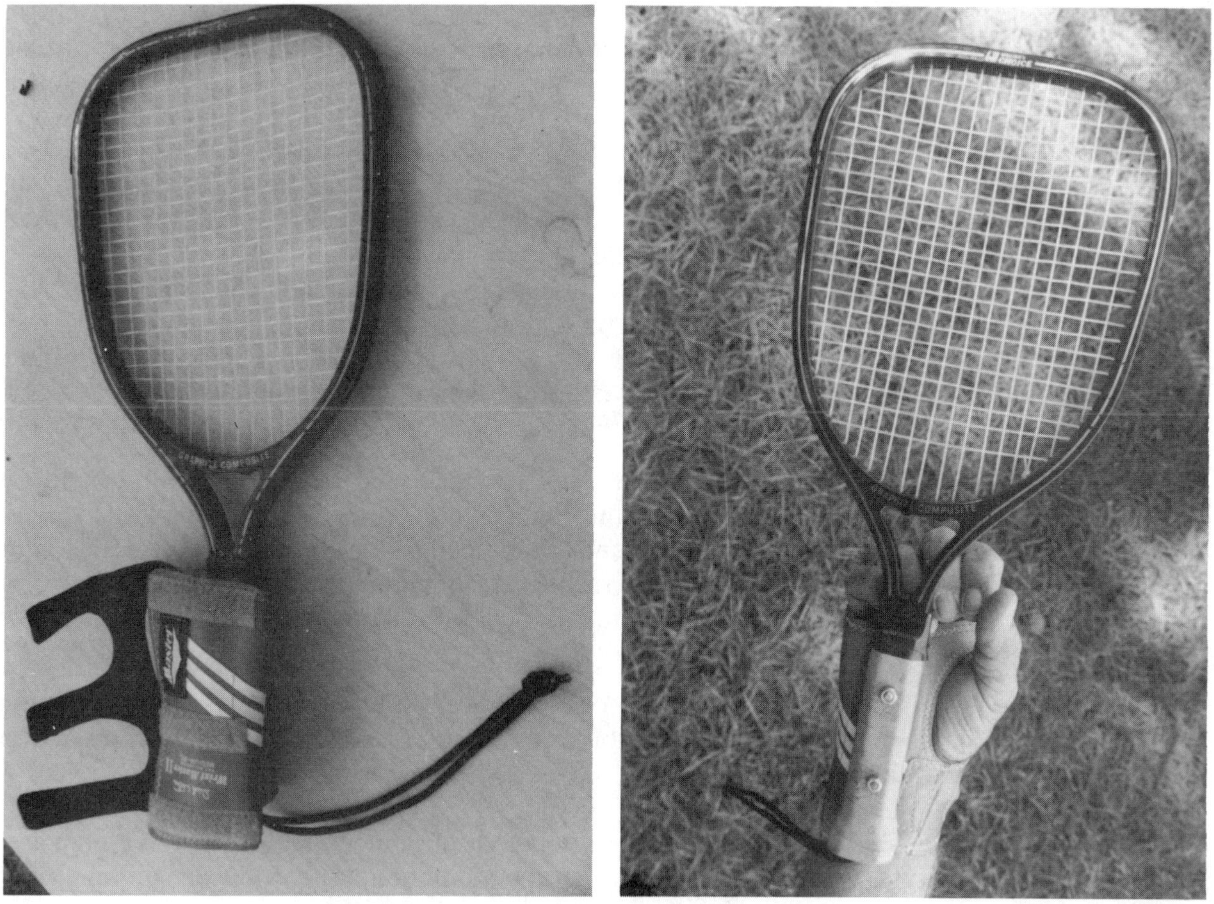

**Figure E–2**: Racquet Ball Racquet — Photograph

3. <u>What you need to build it</u>: The ingredients needed to construct this device are not hard to find. They consist of the following:

   a. One racquet ball racquet.
   b. One bowling glove (left or right handed as indicated).
   c. Two ⅛ inch by 2½ inch bolts and nuts.

4. <u>How you make it</u>: The "recipe" or directions for building this device are as follows:

   a. Place the palm of the bowling glove against the racquet handle.
   b. Mark the position for two holes which will go through both the glove and the racquet handle.
   c. Remove the glove and drill the two holes through the racquet handle.
   d. Place the glove back on the racquet handle and mark the glove to correspond to the site of the two drill holes.
   e. Now drill through glove into the handle's drill holes.
   f. From the glove side, insert the bolts through the glove and handle and attach the nuts to the bolts on the other side of the handle.

5. How it works: The metal bracing inherent in the bowling glove provides the user with the needed wrist support to successfully swing and hit a ball, whether the sport is racquet ball or tennis. The needed hand security is afforded by adjusting the tightness of the Velcro straps, already provided on the bowling glove.

6. Other adaptations: The inherent wrist support afforded by the bowling glove gives the disabled child a great advantage in tennis. Even if tennis is the sport of choice, a racquet ball racquet, rather than a tennis racquet, is suggested to be used due to the long handle of the tennis racquet which would be very heavy and awkward to try to swing effectively. Although the adapted racquet ball racquet system was originally designed to help students play tennis, this bowling glove support/security system can be used for many other sports and skills such as fishing, baseball, golf, badminton, table tennis, etc.

7. Mainstreaming ideas: Since this idea can be used to assist children grasp and effectively use any number of implements (racquets, bats, clubs, etc.) virtually any sport being taught would allow for the successful integration of disabled children, right alongside their able bodied peers, with little or no assistance from anyone, depending upon the degree of their disability.

   a. Populations able to participate: Any students needing wrist support and hand grasping security can participate as both of these needs are provided for by the bowling glove. To participate independently, the student would need to have relatively normal shoulder and elbow function in order to swing the racquet (or implement) effectively. (It is quite possible to be wheelchair bound and utilize this device successfully, as long as reasonable shoulder and elbow function is present).

   b. Examples of use: See numbers 6 through 7a above. Children with cerebral palsy, spinal cord injury, spina myelodysplasia (spina bifida), muscular dystrophy, in most cases, can benefit greatly with this device.

8. Therapeutic benefits: Both national (developmental) and state (curricular) objectives are addressed with this device. Furthermore, therapeutic benefits involving the training of specific muscle groups can be facilitated with the use of this device.

   a. AAHPERD Objectives: This device addresses all five of the AAHPERD Developmental Objectives of Physical Education. See **Figure 1**, Introduction section of this book. Ranked in the conceivable order of their facilitation through this device are:

      1. Neuromuscular: This domain is especially enhanced as the student learns a new sport/lifetime recreational skill.

      2. Emotional: This device will help build self–concept as the student gains in confidence with the knowledge that a new and exciting skill can be learned.

      3. Social: A sense of belonging and acceptance will be fostered as this device will allow the disabled child to join able bodied peers in a multitude of games and sports (especially tennis and racquet ball) that were previously inaccessible. Even the more severely disabled can use this device successfully thus making it an excellent device to have to help integrate disabled children effectively.

      4. Organic: Basic strength, endurance, and flexibility of the shoulder and elbow joints are at least moderately addressed when using this device, even if the child is wheelchair bound. If the child is ambulatory, these organic components of physical fitness are even further developed.

      5. Interpretive: This domain is enhanced as the child learns how to execute the various racquet swings effectively. Just like any other able bodied child, with practice, the

disabled child will learn to place the ball into the opponent's court with the desired speed, spin, direction, etc.

b. State DOE Objectives: This device allows for disabled children to conform to the State DOE (1975) curriculum objectives for physical education; Cluster III (Lifetime Sports); Sections A, and C–F, (Angling, badminton, bowling, fencing, golf, tennis, and paddle ball). See **Figure 2**, Introduction section of this book.

c. Muscle groups trained: The racquet ball racquet directly, or indirectly, addresses all functional muscle groups. If the participant is ambulatory, anti–gravity muscles needed to stand, turn, walk and run are used extensively. These include dorsi and plantar flexors, knee flexors and extensors; hip flexors, extensors, abductors, adductors, and rotators; and trunk flexors, extensors and rotators. If the participant is wheelchair bound, these muscles are used to a lesser extent, depending on the extent of impairment. Both non–ambulatory and ambulatory participants will utilize a combination of all upper extremity muscle groups depending on the phase of the swing (cocking or contact), and depending on the stroke employed.

d. Other information: See #6, "Other Adaptations" above, for a review of other information.

9. Notes:

## F. Tripod Seat

The tripod seat will provide a balance point for physically disabled individuals to experience hitting different balls from a variety of sports including golf, baseball, and racquet sports.

1. Please refer to **Figure F–1** for schematic diagrams which illustrate the construction sequence of this device.

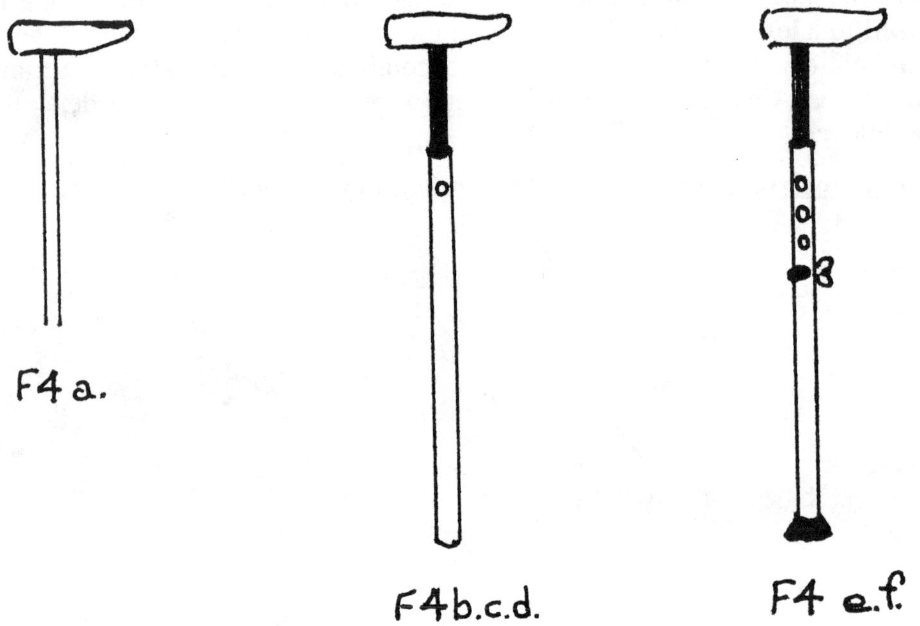


**Figure F–1**: Tripod Seat — Diagram

2. Please refer to **Figure F–2** which are photographs of the tripod seat.

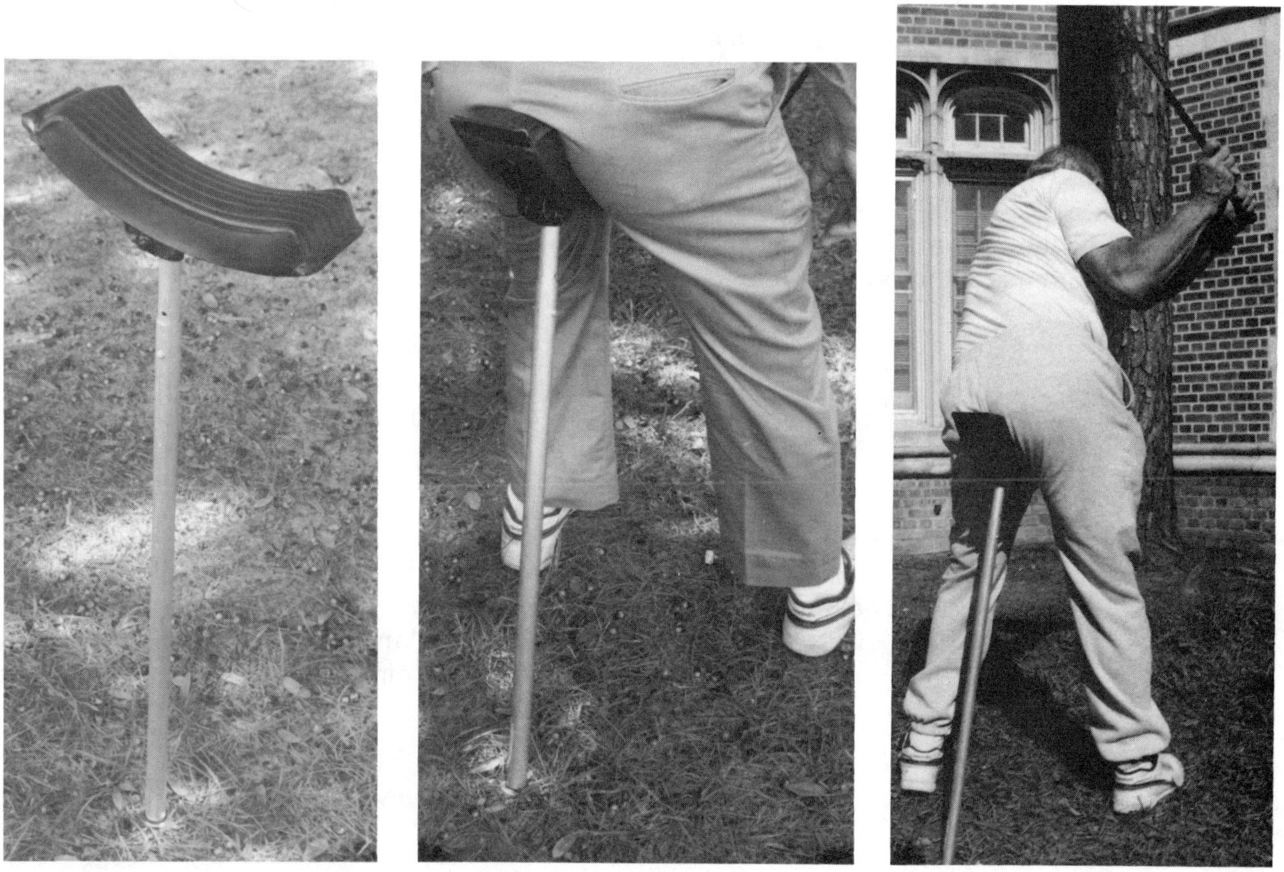

**Figure F–2**: Tripod Seat — Photograph

3. What you need to build it: The ingredients needed to construct this device are not hard to find. They consist of the following:

   a. One bicycle seat.
   b. One piece of 1 inch aluminum tubing two feet long.
   c. One piece of ½ inch aluminum tubing two feet long.
   d. One 1 inch crutch tip.
   e. One ⅛ inch by 1½ inch bolt with wing nut.

4. How to make it: The "recipe" or directions for building this device are as follows:

   a. Attach the bicycle seat to the end of the ½ inch tubing.
   b. Insert clear end of ½ inch tubing into the 1 inch tubing.
   c. Adjust the length of the tubes to make seat at a comfortable height.
   d. Mark and drill a ⅛ inch hole through both tubes.
   e. Secure position with a ⅛ inch by 1½ inch bolt and wing nut.
   f. Drill additional holes in the ½ inch tube at 1 inch intervals (this will allow the seat to be adjustable in height to adapt to users of varying heights.

5. How it works: The seat should be placed in a position where the user can comfortably "sit" on it, while keeping the legs in contact with the ground. This is the "tripod" position. The user can rotate the trunk and actually take the weight off one leg, allowing the seat and the other leg to support the weight of the body. The user can then rotate back the other way through full tripod

contact and continue the rotation through to a two point stance again on the other side. This tripod adaptation allows individuals who cannot stand up and *shift their weight* independently to do so. They can stand and now swing with balance and thus participate in golf, softball, racquet sports, and more, even though they may be dependent on a wheelchair or crutches for normal ambulation.

6. Other adaptations: This sports tripod can be used effectively on various types of surfaces. The rubber crutch tip provides for a stable contact point. If the tripod seat is to be used only on grass, such as for golf, frisbee golf, and other such sports, the crutch tip may be removed and the end of the tubing can be hammered into a pointed tip to insert an inch or so in the grass, which would add even more stability to the device.

7. Mainstreaming ideas: The use of this device will provide the opportunity for any child, who can stand with minimal assistance, to participate alongside his/her able bodied peer, in an effective, successful manner. Once the child attempts a few practice swings, shots, volleys, whatever, with the seat, very little or no further assistance will be needed. The teacher is freed to attend to the rest of the class.

    a. Populations able to participate: Students who normally ambulate with crutches, and some wheelchair students will be able to utilize this device. The student must be able to stand with minimal assistance, and/or, be totally comfortable with the three point tripod position afforded by the standing seat. Children with mild to moderate cerebral palsy, early muscular dystrophy, moderate spinal myelodysplasia (spina bifida; myelomeningocele), incomplete spinal cord injury, and any number of other permanent or temporary disabilities could participate in physical education activities with this device.

    b. Examples of use: See numbers 5 through 7a above for many suggestions for the use of this device.

8. Therapeutic benefits: Both national (developmental) and state (curricular) objectives are addressed with this device. Furthermore, therapeutic benefits involving the training of specific muscle groups can be facilitated with the use of this device.

    a. AAHPERD Objectives: This device addresses all five of the AAHPERD Developmental Objectives of Physical Education. See **Figure 1**, Introduction section of this book. Ranked in the conceivable order of their facilitation through this device are:

        1. Neuromuscular: This domain is enhanced as the student learns new sport/lifetime recreational skills, especially those thought never to be possible. This new found opportunity to stand and shift the body weight in a functional manner demands static and dynamic balance skills as well as non–locomotor skills.

        2. Emotional: This device will help build self–concept as the student gains in confidence with the knowledge that a new and exciting skill can be learned effectively.

        3. Social: A sense of belonging and acceptance will be fostered as this device will allow the disabled child to join able bodied peers in a multitude of games and sports that were previously inaccessible. Even some wheelchair dependent children can use this device successfully thus making it an excellent device to have to help effectively integrate disabled children in physical education.

        4. Organic: Basic strength, endurance, and flexibility of the lower limbs, pelvis, spine and upper limbs are addressed when using this device. This rare opportunity to stand and function with confidence, control, and duration will aid circulation, proprioception, and the maintenance of needed bone density.

5. Interpretive: This domain is enhanced as the child learns how to place the seat to execute the various swings, shots, throws, catches, etc., effectively.

b. State DOE Objectives: This device allows for disabled children to conform to the State DOE (1975) curriculum objectives for physical education; Cluster III (Lifetime Sports); Sections A–C, and F–H (Angling, archery, badminton, golf, tennis, and paddle ball) and Cluster IX, Sections A and B (Active and Quiet Recreational Sports). See **Figure 2**, Introduction section of this book.

c. Muscle groups trained: The sports tripod directly, or indirectly, addresses all functional muscle groups. Anti–gravity muscles needed to stand and rotate the spine are used extensively. Basically, all upper and lower extremity muscles are employed depending on the skill used.

d. Other information: See #6, "Other Adaptations" above, for a review of other information.

9. Notes:

## G. Adapted Baseball/Softball Glove

The adapted glove will provide an opportunity for physically or mentally disabled individuals to catch a ball with confidence.

1. Please refer to **Figure G–1** for schematic diagrams which illustrate the construction sequence of this device.

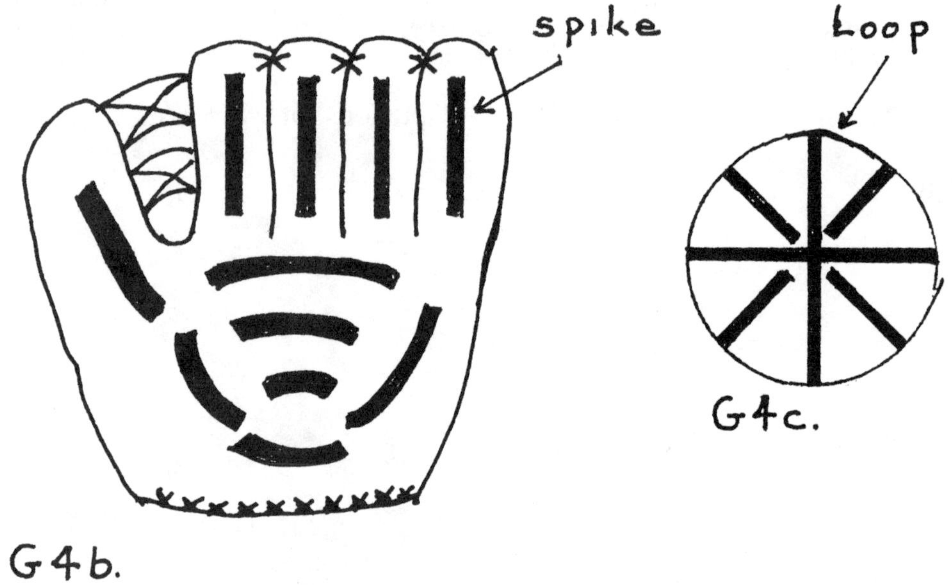


**Figure G–1**: Baseball/Softball Glove — Diagram

2. Please refer to **Figure G–2** which is a photograph of this glove.

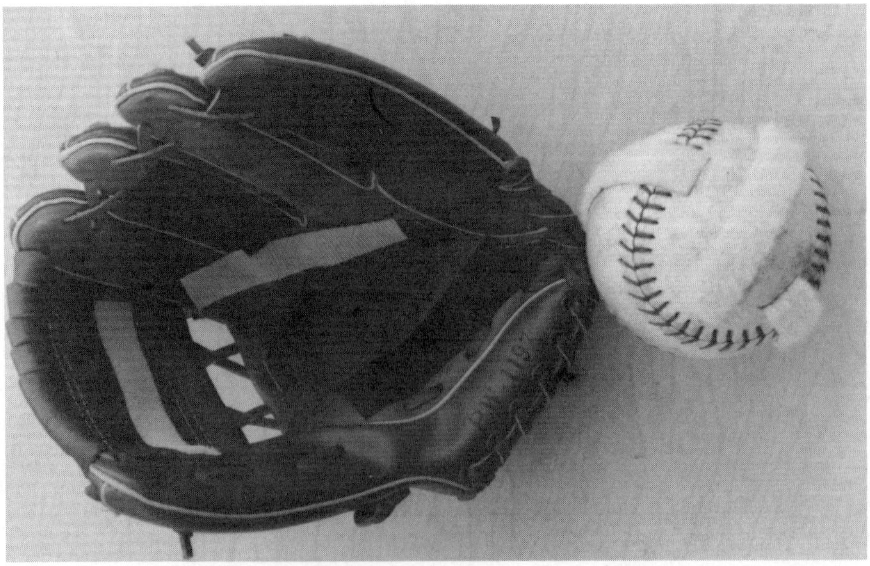

**Figure G–2**: Baseball/Softball Glove — Photograph

3. What you need to build it: The ingredients needed to construct this ball and glove idea are not hard to find. They consist of the following:

   a. One fielder's mitt for baseball or softball.
   b. One 2 foot strip of self–adhesive Velcro.
   c. One baseball or softball.

4. How to make it: The "recipe" or directions for building this device are as follows:

   a. Separate the loop and spike sides of the Velcro.
   b. Using one side of the Velcro, stick the strips to each finger of the glove and three strips across the palm and heel of the glove.
   c. Using the other side of the Velcro, circle the ball with Velcro, then fill in the sides with two strips of velcro.
   d. Now both the ball and the catching surface of the glove should be predominately covered with Velcro.

5. How it works: Since the ball and glove are functionally coated with Velcro strips meant to stick to one another, once the child can get the glove in reasonable proximity to catch the ball, and the ball comes in contact with the strips on the glove, the ball should stick well enough to afford a "catch."

6. Other adaptations: If the baseball or softball are too heavy at first to stick easily to the glove, a lighter ball like a whiffle ball or plastic ball or tennis ball can be used. A lighter weight ball should help children catch little easier until they get the idea and can progress to heavier balls. Also, the amount of Velcro stripping can be increased to literally coat the surface of the ball and glove if further assistance is needed. As the children get more proficient, less stripping is needed.

7. Mainstreaming ideas: The use of this device will provide the opportunity for disabled children to participate in ball skills and games with their able bodied peers with minimal assistance from others. The teacher is more free to attend to the rest of the class.

   a. Populations able to participate: Even the most severely disabled students can "catch" using this idea. If the ball is carefully thrown, even children with no movement or control of their limbs can "catch" the ball. Children with minimal upper extremity function can pick the ball up out of the glove and throw it back to their partners.

   b. Examples of use: See numbers 5 and 6 above for many suggestions for the use of this device.

8. Therapeutic benefits: Both national (developmental) and state (curricular) objectives are addressed with this idea. Furthermore, therapeutic benefits involving the training of specific muscle groups can be facilitated with the use of this ball and glove adaptation.

   a. AAHPERD Objectives: This idea addresses all five of the AAHPERD Developmental Objectives of Physical Education. See **Figure 1**, Introduction section of this book. Ranked in the conceivable order of their facilitation through this device are:

      1. Neuromuscular: This domain is enhanced as the student learns new sport/lifetime recreational skills, especially those thought never to be possible.

      2. Emotional: This idea will help build self–concept as the student gains in confidence with the knowledge that a new and exciting skill can be learned effectively.

3. Social: A sense of belonging and acceptance will be fostered as this ball and glove idea will allow the disabled child to join able bodied peers in a multitude of games and sports that were previously inaccessible. Even some wheelchair dependent children can use this device successfully thus making it an excellent device to have to help effectively integrate disabled children in physical education.

4. Organic: Basic strength, endurance, and especially flexibility of the upper limbs are addressed when using this idea.

5. Interpretive: This domain is enhanced as the child learns how to anticipate the direction of throws and actually catch a ball. State DOE Objectives: This idea allows for disabled children to conform to the State DOE (1975) curriculum objectives for physical education; Cluster IV (Team Games); and Cluster IX, Sections A and B (Active and Quiet Recreational Sports). See **Figure 2**, Introduction section of this book.

b. Muscle groups trained: The adapted ball and glove idea helps to directly address all functional muscle groups of the upper extremities; and indirectly, all other muscle groups of the body if the child is ambulatory and can therefore "catch and throw on the move."

9. Notes:

## H. Adapted Throwing Glove

The adapted throwing glove will provide an opportunity for physically disabled individuals (especially those with hypertonicity) to successfully throw a ball.

1. Please refer to **Figure H–1** for schematic diagrams which illustrate the construction sequence of this device.

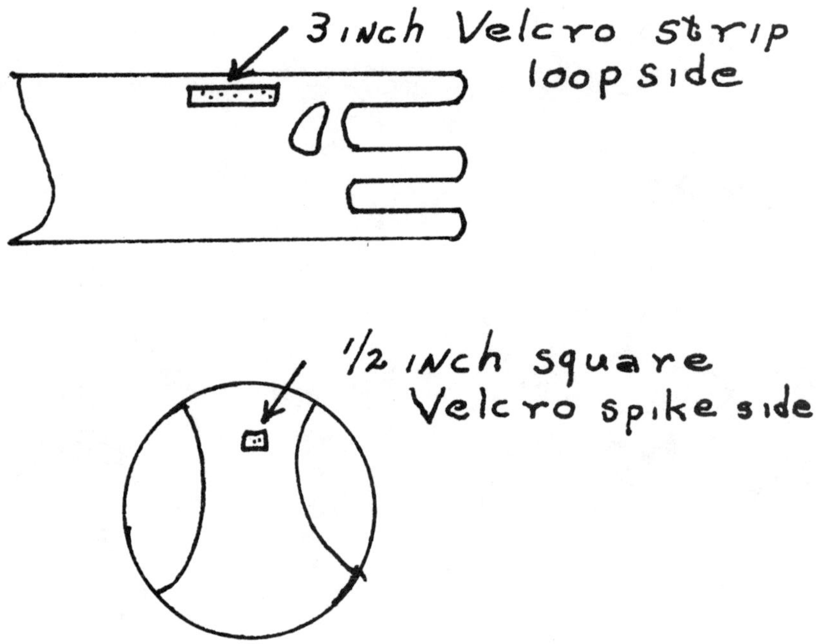


**Figure H–1**: Adapted Throwing Glove — Diagram

2. Please refer to **Figure H–2** which are photographs of this glove.

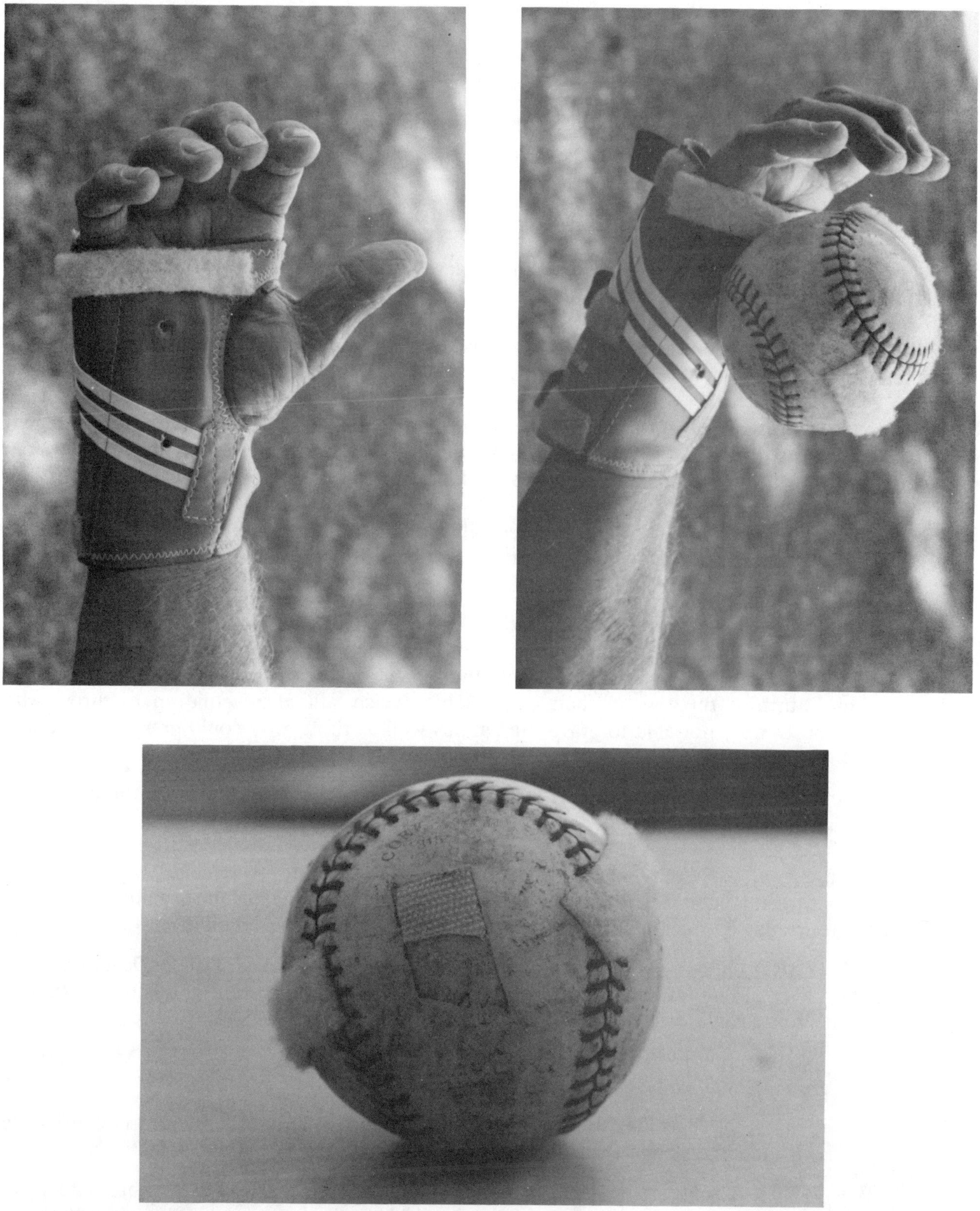

**Figure H–2**: Adapted Throwing Glove — Photograph

3. What you need to build it: The ingredients needed to construct this glove are not hard to find. They consist of the following:

   a. One bowling glove (right or left hand).
   b. One 3 inch strip of Velcro (loop side).
   c. One ½ inch square of Velcro (spike side).

4. How to make it: The "recipe" or directions for building this device are as follows:

   a. Stick the loop side strip of Velcro to the bowling glove. Position the strip at the base of the fingers.
   b. Stick the ½ inch square piece of Velcro to a ball such as a softball.

5. How it works: Since the ball and glove have Velcro strips meant to stick to each another, the child (or an assistant) simply places the ball in the bowling glove, cocks the ball and glove unit back as able, and performs the best approximation of a throwing motion. The acceleration coupled with the sudden deceleration at the end of the throwing motion will allow the ball to release itself from grasp of the Velcro strips.

6. Other adaptations: If the softball is too heavy at first to stick easily to the glove, a lighter ball like a whiffle ball or plastic ball or tennis ball can be used. A lighter weight ball may help children throw a little easier until they get the idea and can progress to heavier balls.

7. Mainstreaming ideas: The use of this device will provide the opportunity for disabled children to participate in ball skills and games with their able bodied peers with minimal assistance from others. The teacher is more free to attend to the rest of the class.

   a. Populations able to participate: Even the most severely disabled students can "throw" using this idea. Children with minimal upper extremity function can use the previously discussed adapted fielder's glove to catch the ball; then, they can use this throwing glove to assist in their returning the toss to their peers. This device will allow children to throw who previously were not able to grasp the ball, as well as those who could grasp it, but could not release it at the proper time to throw, or at all.

   b. Examples of use: See numbers 5 through 7a above for many suggestions for the use of this device.

8. Therapeutic benefits: Both national (developmental) and state (curricular) objectives are addressed with this idea. Furthermore, therapeutic benefits involving the training of specific muscle groups can be facilitated with the use of this ball and glove adaptation.

   a. AAHPERD Objectives: This idea addresses all five of the AAHPERD Developmental Objectives of Physical Education. See **Figure 1**, Introduction section of this book. Ranked in the conceivable order of their facilitation through this device are:

      1. Neuromuscular: This domain is enhanced as the student learns new sport/lifetime recreational skills, especially those thought never to be possible.

      2. Emotional: This idea will help build self–concept as the student gains in confidence with the knowledge that a new and exciting skill can be learned effectively.

      3. Social: A sense of belonging and acceptance will be fostered as this ball and glove idea will allow the disabled child to join able bodied peers in a multitude of games and sports that were previously inaccessible. Even some wheelchair dependent children can use this device successfully thus making it an excellent device to have to help effectively integrate disabled children in physical education.

4. Organic: Basic strength, endurance, and especially flexibility of the upper limbs are addressed when using this idea.

5. Interpretive: This domain is enhanced as the child learns how to aim for a target in regard to direction and distance and actually throw a ball successfully.

b. State DOE Objectives: This idea allows for disabled children to conform to the State DOE (1975) curriculum objectives for physical education; Cluster IV (Team Games); and Cluster IX, Sections A and B (Active and Quiet Recreational Sports). See **Figure 2**, Introduction section of this book.

c. Muscle groups trained: This adapted throwing glove idea helps to directly address all functional muscle groups of the upper extremities; and indirectly, all other muscle groups of the body if the child is ambulatory and can therefore "throw" while running.

d. Other information: See #6, "Other Adaptations" above, for a review of other information.

9. Notes:

## I. Adapted Swim Fin

The adapted swim fin will provide an opportunity for amputees to swim with a balanced and symmetrical arm stroke or kick.

1. Please refer to **Figure I–1** for schematic diagrams which illustrate the construction sequence of this device.

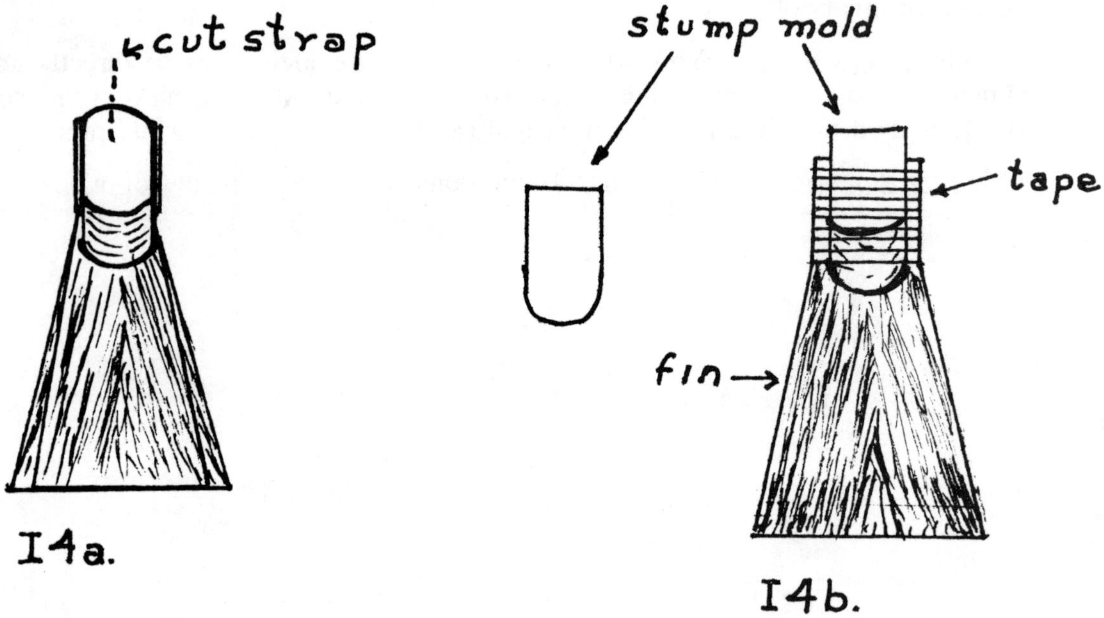


**Figure I–1**: Adapted Swim Fin — Diagram

2. Please refer to **Figure I–2** which are photographs of this adapted fin.

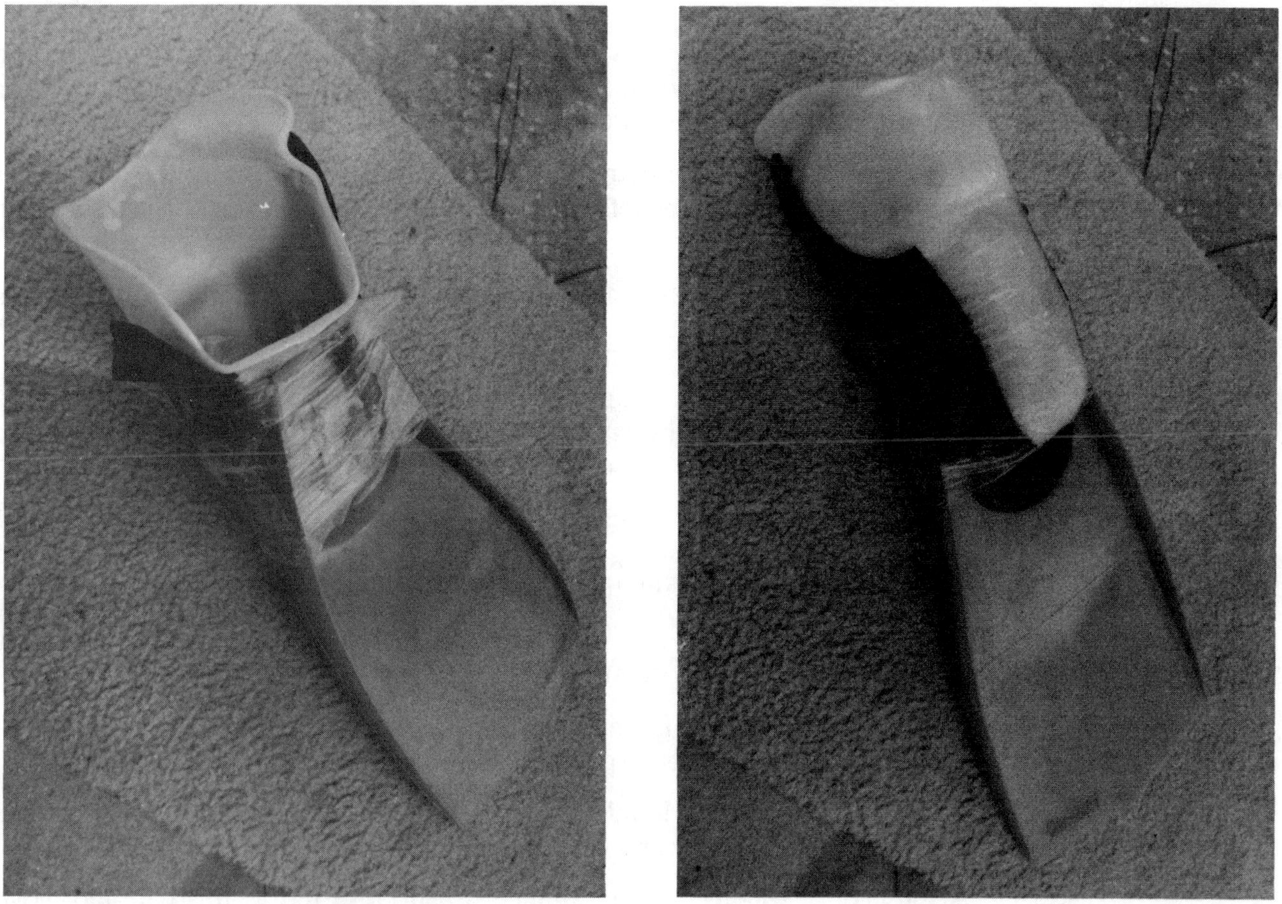

**Figure I–2**: Adapted Swim Fin — Photograph

3. What you need to build it: The ingredients needed to construct this fin are not hard to find. They consist of the following:
   a. One set of swim fins.
   b. One roll of waterproof tape.
   c. One extra mold of the disabled limb's stump. (Have the prosthetist who makes the person's prosthesis make an extra mold of the stump.)

4. How to make it: The "recipe" or directions for building this device are as follows:
   a. Split the heel section of the fin and pull the fin foot section as far over the mold as possible.
   b. As tightly as possible, wrap water proof tape around the mold and swim fin.

5. How it works: People with amputations of the lower limb often find it difficult to swim efficiently without the other leg to serve as a rudder and to a very limited extent, a minor propulsion unit, as legs normally do with able bodied swimmers. To prevent unequal drag forces and to reclaim the balance, stability, and minor propulsion missing from an amputee, the use of this adapted swim fin is highly recommended. Of course, the wearer should use the matching fin on the other "good" leg's foot.

6. Other adaptations: It is effective for both above knee and below knee amputees. It is easily slipped on and worn comfortably for the entire workout. The size and weight of the fin should be selected in accordance with the disabled person's size and strength. Obviously, larger, stronger people will need larger, heavier fins than smaller, lighter people.

7. Mainstreaming ideas: The use of this device will provide the opportunity for disabled children to participate in aquatic skills units with their able bodied peers with minimal assistance from others. The teacher is more free to attend to the rest of the class.

   a. Populations able to participate: Other than amputees, hemiplegics and others needing lower extremity control or buoyancy may benefit from wearing an appropriately sized swim fin to one or both feet.

   b. Examples of use: See numbers 5 through 7a above for suggestions for the use of this device.

8. Therapeutic benefits: Both national (developmental) and state (curricular) objectives are addressed with this idea. Furthermore, therapeutic benefits involving the training of specific muscle groups can be facilitated with the use of this adapted swim fin idea.

   a. AAHPERD Objectives: This idea addresses all five of the AAHPERD Developmental Objectives of Physical Education. See **Figure 1,** Introduction section of this book. Ranked in the conceivable order of their facilitation through this device are:

      1. Organic: Strength, endurance, and flexibility are all especially enhanced with they ability to swim laps efficiently, due to this device.

      2. Neuromuscular: This domain is enhanced as the student learns new aquatic and sport/lifetime recreational skills, especially those thought never to be possible.

      3. Emotional: This idea will help build self–concept as the student gains in confidence with the knowledge that a new and exciting skill can be learned effectively.

      4. Social: A sense of belonging and acceptance will be fostered as this ball and glove idea will allow the disabled child to join able bodied peers in a multitude of games and sports that were previously inaccessible. Even wheelchair dependent children can often use this swim fin idea successfully thus making it an excellent device to have to help effectively integrate disabled children in physical education.

      5. Interpretive: This domain is enhanced as the child is now able to learn new strokes and practice them to perfection.

   b. State DOE Objectives: This idea allows for disabled children to conform to the State DOE (1975) curriculum objectives for physical education; Cluster VIII (Aquatics) Sections A–D, especially B (Swimming). See **Figure 2,** Introduction section of this book.

   c. Muscle groups trained: This adapted swimming fin helps to directly address all working muscle groups of the entire body.

   d. Other information: See #6, "Other Adaptations" above, for a review of other information.

9. Notes:

# PART TWO:

**Miscellaneous Ideas**
**(all of which can be home–made, or are very affordable)**

## General Concepts

When disabilities are present, it follows that modifications in equipment are necessary. Adaptive equipment is used to help individuals overcome obstacles inherent to their disability. When used appropriately, adaptive equipment can facilitate the fulfillment needed physical education objectives. Personal satisfaction and success become a reality.

Adaptive equipment does not have to be complicated or expensive in order to achieve these goals. Simple equipment modifications can help to prevent failure and increase successful and enjoyable experiences. The frequency and degree to which this is true is dependent on the creativity and experience of the individuals involved.

The tables in this section list various types of equipment ideas. Physical education objectives are listed across the top left of each table. The •'s denote where the equipment idea can in some way be used to *help address a physical education objective*. In addition, various special population groups are listed across the top right of each table. The +'s are found where an equipment idea is *recommended* for a particular special population. The —'s denote where the idea is *contraindicated* for reasons of physical demand, safety, or sophistication. In several instances, the equipment idea received a — because it was too simplistic, or too unchallenging for the population concerned. Finally, o's indicate where the equipment idea *may or may not* be recommended depending on the severity of the child's disability, stage of his particular progressive disease, and the specific modifications incorporated into the activity itself.

Basically, the idea is to initially glance at the table as a whole unit. Notice on the left hand side that there are many more "filled in" places than there are "blanks." This implies the potential available from the possible adaptations of everyday equipment. Clearly, all children should be involved in physical education activities. If the specific activity is not contraindicated for the child's particular condition, significant benefit would seem inevitable. An important implication of this table is that most all activities are recommended for all special population groups. Although priorities may be variable, all objectives of physical education are indicated for all special populations.

1. ROPES: The various uses of ropes are extensive. See **Table 1** (Page 41).
   a. Rope skipping — Ropes can be skipped independently, or with a group; overhead/sagittal plane, or circular/transverse plane.
   b. Tug of war — This can be played by conventional two team action, or, tie each team rope to a center circle of rope, symmetrically. When tension is applied, the center rope section becomes a triangle, or a square, or a pentagon, etc., depending on the number of team ropes pulling. See **Figure 3**.

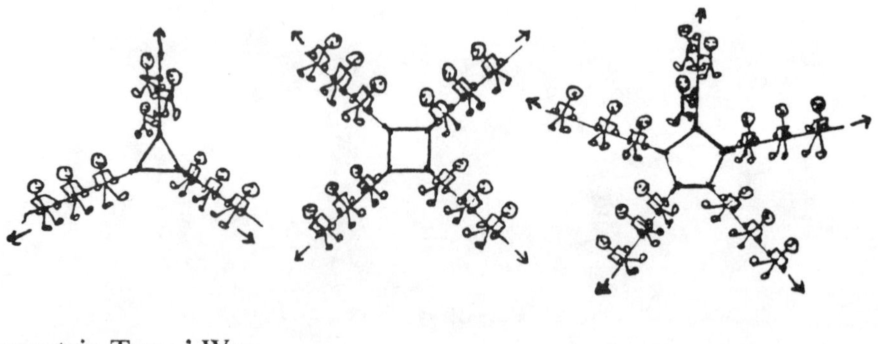

**Figure 3**: Geometric Tug o' War

| Ropes | ORGANIC | | | | NEUROMUSCULAR—PERCEPTUAL MOTOR | | | | | | | | | | | | | | | | | | | | | | | INTERPRETIVE | SOCIO–EMOTIONAL |
|---|---|---|---|---|---|---|---|---|---|---|---|---|---|---|---|---|---|---|---|---|---|---|---|---|---|---|---|---|---|
| | Strength | Endurance | Flexibility | Relaxation | Motor Factors — | Coordination | Agility | Power | Rhythm | Developmental — | Inappropriate reflex inhibition; normal reaction facilitation | Gross Motor: locomotor skills | Gross Motor: nonlocomotor skills | Fine Motor: Prehension and manipulative skills | Sensori–Motor control | Eye–hand/foot | Ear–hand/foot | Receipt–propulsion | Kinesthesia | Proprioception | Laterality | Directionality | Spatial Awareness | Balance — | Static | Dynamic | Vestibular | | |
| Rope skipping | | • | | | | • | • | • | • | | • | • | | | | • | • | | • | • | • | • | • | | | • | | • | • |
| Tug of war | • | • | | | | • | | • | • | | • | | • | • | | • | • | | • | • | | | | | • | • | | • | • |
| Balance Skills intro. | | | | | | • | | | | | • | • | | | | • | | | • | • | • | • | • | | • | • | | • | • |
| Spotting belts | | | • | • | | • | | • | | | • | • | • | | | • | • | | • | • | • | • | • | | • | • | • | • | • |
| Obstacles | • | | • | | | • | • | • | • | | • | • | • | | | • | | | • | • | • | • | • | | • | • | | • | • |
| Movement exploration | • | • | • | • | | • | • | • | • | | • | • | • | • | | • | • | • | • | • | • | • | • | | • | • | • | • | • |
| Rope ladders | • | • | • | | | • | • | • | • | | • | • | • | • | | • | | | • | • | • | • | • | | • | • | • | • | • |
| Tetherball games | | | | | | • | • | • | • | | • | | • | • | | • | • | • | • | • | • | • | • | | • | | | • | • |
| Return lines | | | | • | | • | | | | | | | • | • | | • | | • | | | | • | • | | | | | • | • |
| Ring–string ball jump | | • | | | | • | • | | • | | • | • | | | | • | | | • | • | • | • | • | | • | • | | • | • |
| Fine motor rope play | | | • | • | | • | | | | | • | | | • | | • | | | • | • | | | • | | | | | • | • |
| Stilts | | • | | | | • | • | | • | | • | • | | | | • | | | • | • | • | • | • | | • | • | | • | • |
| Swings | • | • | • | • | | • | • | • | • | | • | | • | • | | • | | • | • | • | • | • | • | | • | • | • | • | • |

| Ropes | PHYSICAL DISABILITIES | | | | | | | | | | | MEDICAL | | | | | | SENSORY | | | | | | | | | |
|---|---|---|---|---|---|---|---|---|---|---|---|---|---|---|---|---|---|---|---|---|---|---|---|---|---|---|---|
| | Spinal Cord Injury | Spinal Myelodysplasia | Amputations | Cerebral Palsy | Muscular Dystropy | Arthritis, arthegryposia, osteogenesis imperfecta | Temporary Conditions — | Fractures | Scoliosis, Kyphosis, Lordosis | Legg–Parthes Disease | Slipped capital Femoral Epiphysis | Diabetes | Cystic Fibrosis | Luekemia | Epilepsy | Hemophilia | Ostomies | Visually Impaired | Hearing Impaired | Developmental Delay | Clumsy Child | Educable MR | Trainable MR | Severe/profound MR | LEARNING DISABILITIES | EMOTIONALLY DISTURBED | SENIOR CITIZENS |
| Rope skipping | — | — | o | o | o | o | — | — | o | — | — | + | + | + | + | + | + | + | + | + | + | + | + | + | + | + | + |
| Tug of war | + | + | + | + | + | + | — | — | o | o | o | + | + | + | + | + | + | + | + | + | + | + | + | + | + | + | + |
| Balance Skills intro. | o | + | + | + | o | + | o | o | + | + | + | + | + | + | + | + | + | o | + | + | + | + | + | + | + | + | + |
| Spotting belts | o | o | + | o | o | + | — | — | + | — | — | + | + | + | o | o | o | + | + | + | + | + | + | + | + | + | + |
| Obstacles | o | o | o | o | o | o | o | o | + | o | o | + | + | + | + | + | + | + | + | + | + | + | + | + | + | + | + |
| Movement exploration | + | + | + | + | + | + | + | + | + | + | + | + | + | + | + | + | + | + | + | + | + | + | + | + | + | + | + |
| Rope ladders | o | o | + | + | o | + | o | o | + | — | — | + | + | + | + | + | + | + | + | + | + | + | + | + | + | + | + |
| Tetherball games | + | + | + | + | + | + | + | + | + | + | + | + | + | + | + | + | + | + | + | + | + | + | + | + | + | + | + |
| Return lines | + | + | + | + | + | + | + | + | + | + | + | + | + | + | + | + | + | + | + | + | + | + | + | + | + | + | + |
| Ring–string ball jump | — | — | o | o | o | o | o | o | o | — | — | + | + | + | + | + | + | + | + | + | + | + | + | + | + | + | + |
| Fine motor rope play | + | + | + | + | + | + | + | + | + | + | + | + | + | + | + | + | + | + | + | + | + | + | + | + | + | + | + |
| Stilts | — | — | — | — | — | o | — | — | o | — | — | + | + | + | + | — | + | o | + | + | + | + | o | — | + | o | o |
| Swings | o | o | + | o | o | o | — | — | + | + | + | + | + | + | o | + | + | + | + | + | + | + | + | + | + | + | + |

**Table 1**: Ideas with Ropes

c. Balance skills introduction — Ropes may be placed rather wide apart and somewhat parallel for the child to learn to stay within while walking. Gradually narrow the ropes to feed the child onto lines on the floor or onto planks, and finally onto low, stable balance beams. Make the ropes form a rather tortuous path, so when the child walks on to the floor line, plank or beam, the mastering of these becomes quite easy. See **Figures 4 and 5**.

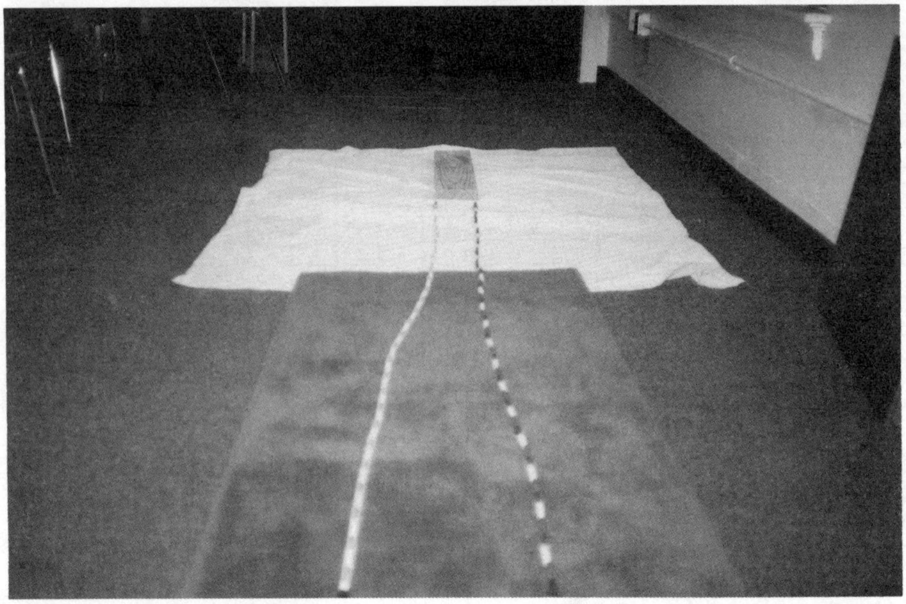

**Figure 4**: Beginning Balance

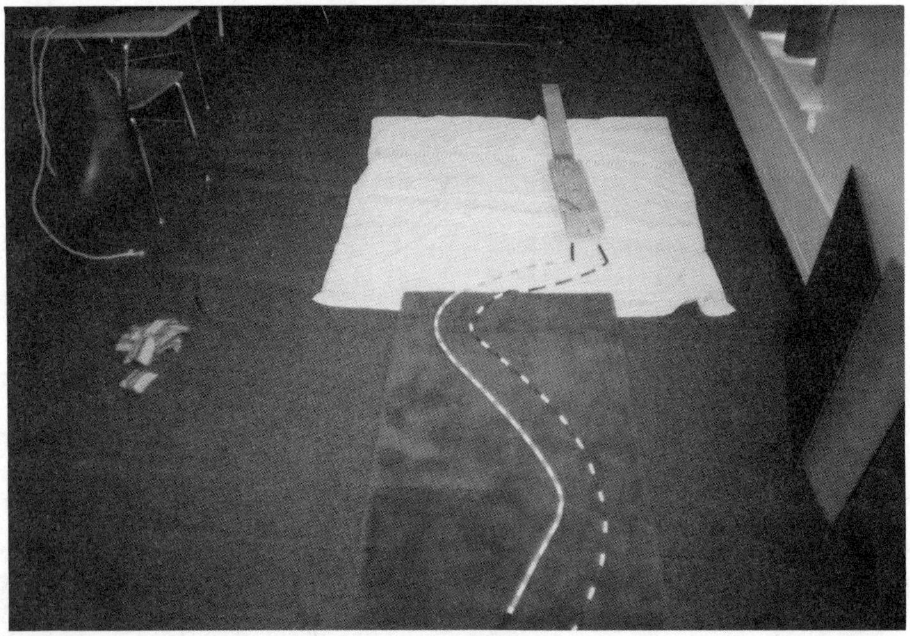

**Figure 5**: Intermediate Balance

d. Spotting belts — With small children, light weight ropes can be used very effectively in providing further security to a safe and carefully supervised tumbling or trampoline unit. A 4 by 6 inch cloth remnant also can be used, especially for larger children. See **Figure 6**.

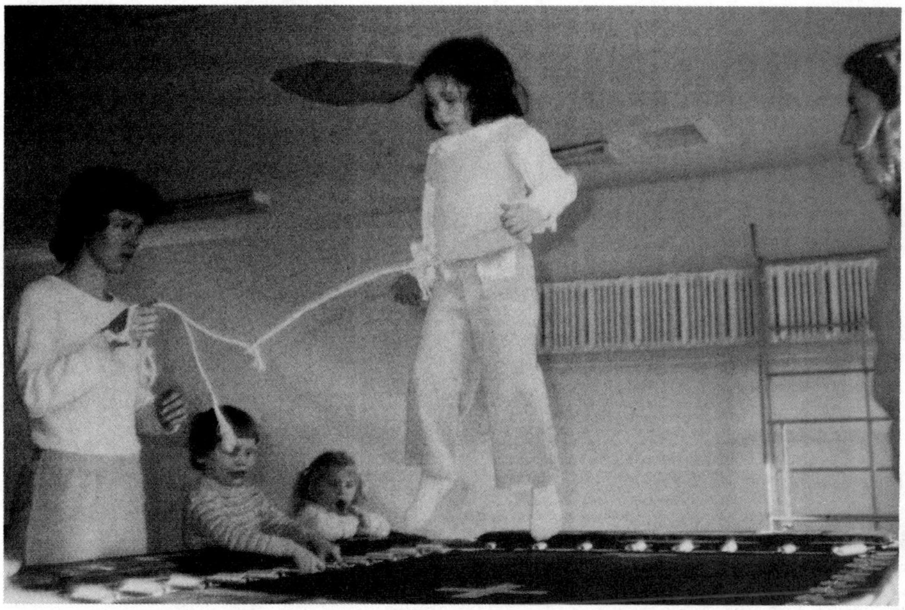

**Figure 6**: Spotting Belt

e. Obstacles — Strung across cones, chairs, etc., ropes can be high jumped, rolled over, rolled under, crawled under, "limbo'd", and more. Balls can be tossed, kicked, or hit into the "rope" designated target areas.

f. Movement exploration — Experiences here are limitless. A small rope can be given to each child and commands given in an exploratory fashion, e.g., "Can you make a box with your rope and fit your whole body inside?" Also, have children, individually or in groups, form letters, words, numbers, and geometric shapes with their groups.

g. Rope ladders — With only three to seven drilled dowels, depending on preferences of length, ropes can be strung through and knotted to easily create an exciting and fitness-stimulating rope ladder. Hang these ladders from the wall, ceiling, or simply suspend them from another climbing apparatus to ensure a close, safe, and matted landing. See **Figure 7**.

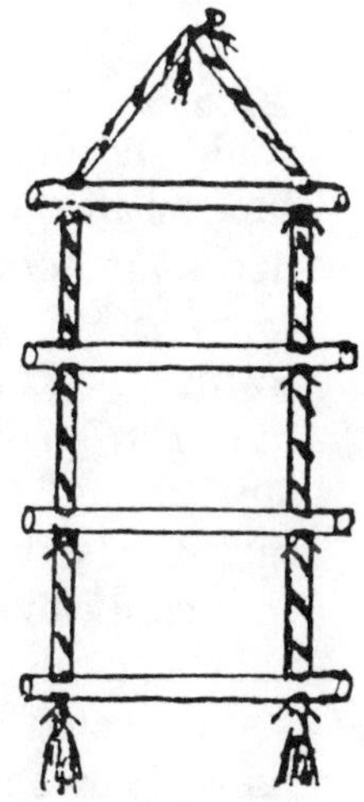

**Figure 7**: Rope Ladder

h. Tetherball games — Ropes can be tied to balls and poles to form tetherball games, from large regulation sizes down to more portable sizes, even table sizes. See **Figure 8**.

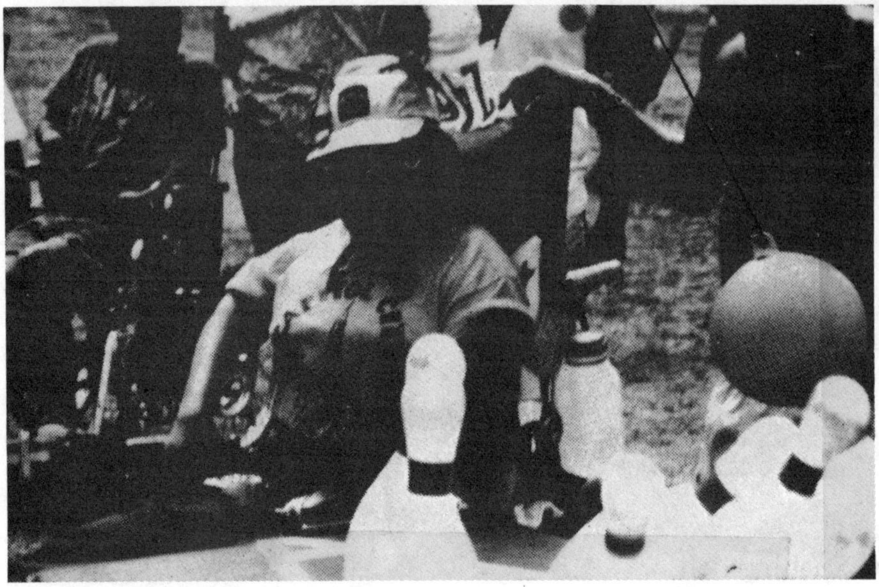

**Figure 8**: Table Tetherball

i. Return lines — Strings attached to whiffle balls and ping–pong balls are a help in eliminating the problems of ball retrieval, especially for the blind, aged, emotionally disturbed, or severely physically handicapped.

j. Ring–a–string ball jump — Use a rubber ring, or cut about 19 inches of garden hose and tape to a circle. If the ends are joined to a small dowel it is easier to form the ring. Then, tape a 2 to 3 foot string from the ring to a little ball. Insert the child's foot through the ring. Now instruct the child to get the ball circling around the ankle by jumping the ball and string on each pass with the other foot. Once the basic skill is learned, the fun can be enhanced with dance rhythms to music, etc.

k. Fine motor rope work — Simply balling up, tying, untying, braiding, and knotting rope will help improve fine motor strength, dexterity, and control.

l. Stilts — Rope and "coffee can" stilts should not be forgotten. These require and enhance static and dynamic balance, motor planning and motor control. This easy to make idea is fun for all ages. Be sure to carefully "spot" children who are new to this or who lack the necessary coordination; success, not injury, is the goal.

m. Swings — Ropes can be used both *for* and *as* swings, climbing ropes, Tarzan vines, and more. In **Figure 9**, two jump ropes are hung from a standard playground pull–up bar. A small board (e.g., an 18 inch 2 by 4) is inserted into the looped ends of the ropes. In a matter of seconds, a portable, safe (if directly supervised), and effective swing is constructed for small children. Where drills and saws are available, a versatile one rope circular swing can be easily constructed. See **Figure 10**. With the addition of a few dowels, a rather sophisticated vestibular swing is possible. See **Figure 11**. One to four ropes can used for hanging tires in various ways. If a net is available, a hammock swing can be easily devised. These are safe, therapeutic, and very enjoyable, even for the severely physically disabled.

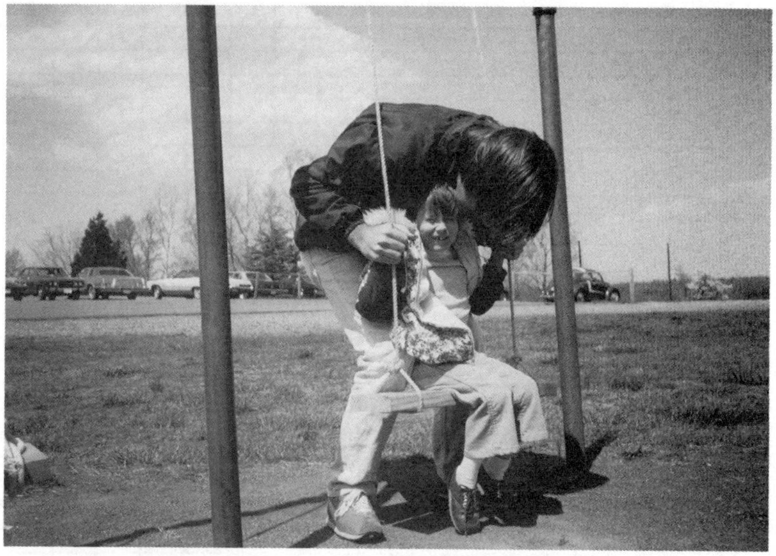

**Figure 9**: Instant Swing

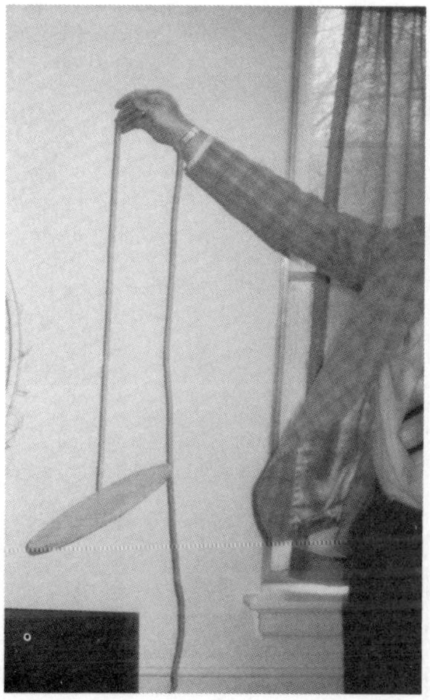

**Figure 10**: Single Rope Swing

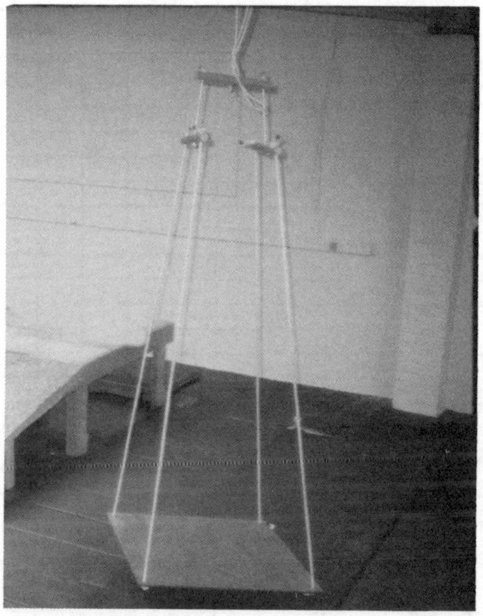

**Figure 11**: Vestibular Swing

2. <u>BOARDS</u>: As with ropes, the various uses of boards appear limited only by a person's ingenuity. See **Table 2** (Page 46).

   a. <u>Steps</u> — For example, adjacent boards stacked at varying heights can be used to promote stair climbing skills, in fearful developmentally delayed children. See **Figure 12**.

**Table 2**: Boards

| Boards | Strength (ORGANIC) | Endurance (ORGANIC) | Flexibility (ORGANIC) | Relaxation (ORGANIC) | Motor Factors — (NEUROMUSCULAR—PERCEPTUAL MOTOR) | Coordination | Agility | Power | Rhythm | Developmental — | Inappropriate reflex inhibition; normal reaction facilitation | Gross Motor: locomotor skills | Gross Motor: nonlocomotor skills | Fine Motor: Prehension and manipulative skills | Sensori-Motor control | Eye-hand/foot | Ear-hand/foot | Receipt-propulsion | Kinesthesia | Proprioception | Laterality | Directionality | Spatial Awareness | Balance — | Static | Dynamic | Vestibular | INTERPRETIVE | SOCIO-EMOTIONAL | |
|---|---|---|---|---|---|---|---|---|---|---|---|---|---|---|---|---|---|---|---|---|---|---|---|---|---|---|---|---|---|---|
| Steps | | | | | | • | • | • | • | | • | • | | | | • | | | • | • | | • | • | | • | • | | • | • | |
| Stepping stones | | | • | | | • | • | • | • | | • | • | | | | • | | | • | • | • | • | • | | • | • | | • | • | |
| Balance boards | | • | | | | • | | | • | | • | | • | | | • | | | • | • | • | • | • | | • | | • | • | • | |
| Bounce boards | • | • | | • | | • | • | • | • | | • | • | • | | | • | • | | • | • | • | • | • | | • | • | • | • | • | |
| Scooter boards | • | • | • | • | | • | • | • | • | | • | • | • | | | • | | | • | • | • | • | • | | • | • | • | • | • | |
| Balance beams | • | | • | | | • | • | • | • | | • | • | • | | | • | | | • | • | • | • | • | | • | • | • | • | • | |
| Slides and planes | | | | • | | • | | | | | • | • | | | | • | | • | • | • | • | • | • | | • | • | • | • | • | |
| See-saws | • | • | • | • | | • | • | • | • | | • | | • | | | • | | | • | • | • | • | • | | • | • | • | • | • | |
| Bowling ramps | | | | • | | • | | | | | • | | | • | | • | | • | • | • | • | • | • | | | | | • | • | |
| Adapted ping-pong | | | | • | | • | | | • | | • | | • | • | | • | • | • | • | • | • | • | • | | • | • | | • | • | |

| Boards | Spinal Cord Injury (PHYSICAL DISABILITIES) | Spinal Myelodysplasia | Amputations | Cerebral Palsy | Muscular Dystropy | Arthritis, arthegryposia, osteogenesis imperfecta | Temporary Conditions — | Fractures | Scoliosis, Kyphosis, Lordosis | Legg-Parthes Disease | Slipped capital Femoral Epiphysis | Diabetes (MEDICAL) | Cystic Fibrosis | Luekemia | Epilepsy | Hemophilia | Ostomies | Visually Impaired (SENSORY) | Hearing Impaired (SENSORY) | Developmental Delay | Clumsy Child | Educable MR | Trainable MR | Severe/profound MR | LEARNING DISABILITIES | EMOTIONALLY DISTURBED | SENIOR CITIZENS |
|---|---|---|---|---|---|---|---|---|---|---|---|---|---|---|---|---|---|---|---|---|---|---|---|---|---|---|---|
| Steps | o | o | + | + | o | + | o | o | + | o | o | + | + | + | + | + | + | + | + | + | + | | | | | | |
| Stepping stones | o | o | + | o | o | o | o | o | + | + | + | + | + | + | + | + | + | o | + | + | + | + | + | + | + | + | + |
| Balance boards | o | o | + | o | + | o | o | o | + | + | + | + | + | + | + | + | + | + | + | + | + | + | + | + | + | + | + |
| Bounce boards | o | o | + | o | o | o | o | o | — | — | — | + | + | + | o | o | + | + | + | + | + | + | + | + | + | + | + |
| Scooter boards | o | o | + | o | o | o | o | o | + | o | o | + | + | + | + | + | + | + | + | + | + | + | + | + | + | + | + |
| Balance beams | o | o | + | o | o | o | o | o | + | o | o | + | + | + | + | + | + | + | + | + | + | + | + | + | + | + | + |
| Slides and planes | o | o | + | o | o | o | o | o | + | o | o | + | + | + | + | o | + | + | + | + | + | + | + | + | + | + | + |
| See-saws | — | o | + | o | o | o | o | o | + | o | o | + | + | + | + | + | + | + | + | + | + | + | + | + | + | + | + |
| Bowling ramps | + | + | + | + | + | + | + | + | — | o | o | — | o | o | o | o | — | + | — | + | + | — | + | + | — | o | o |
| Adapted ping-pong | + | + | + | + | + | + | + | + | — | + | + | o | o | o | o | o | — | + | — | + | + | — | + | + | — | o | o |

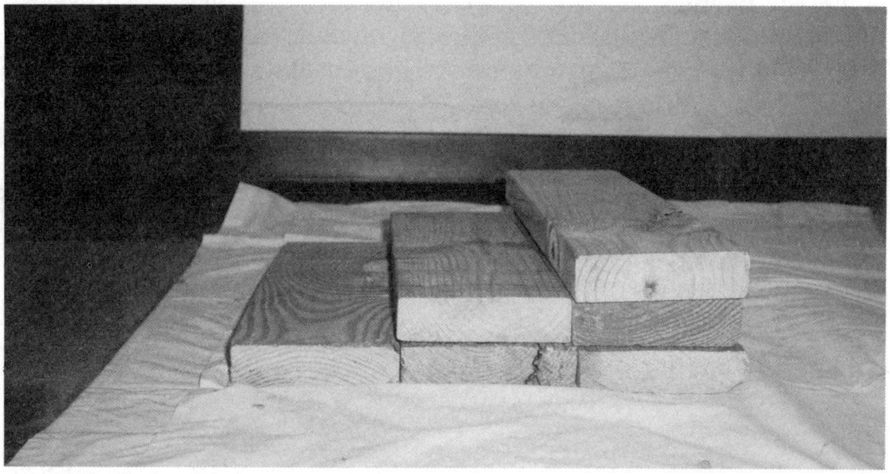

**Figure 12**: Lead–up Steps

b. Stepping stones — Small boards (approximately 12 by 12 inches) can be spaced along the floor for the child to move along like stepping stones. This activity especially helps laterality, directionality, balance, sequencing, and coordination of body parts. Foot steps can be applied to these "stones" and various colors and numbers added to further stimulate interpretive development.

c. Balance boards — These can be constructed by nailing a block or dowel to the bottom of a board. The larger the block or dowel, the more difficult it is to balance. So, several boards can be utilized to provide for a larger range of balance demands. See **Figure 13**.

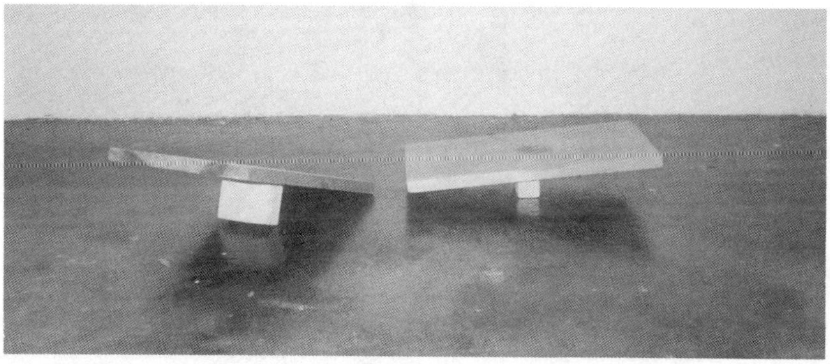

**Figure 13**: Balance Boards

d. Bounce Boards — A plank set across two tires creates a very simple and effective bouncing board. The size of the tires, board, and child will dictate the amount of elasticity, or bounce, that the board will produce.

e. Balance beam — A balance beam can be securely constructed by placing two approximately 10 foot long 2 by 4's to each other, parallel, up on edge, so that the 2 inch sides are facing up and down. Two additional 2 by 4's, each about 2 feet long, should be nailed in a perpendicular direction, about 15 inches from each end, to serve as legs to support the beam off the floor. These legs provide stability to the beam to prevent it from tipping over.

See **Figures 14a–c**. Beam skills can be easily mastered when sufficient instruction in lead–up skills is provided. These lead up skills my include static standing positions on the floor then beam, and floor to beam walking forward, backward, sideways, with turns, over obstacles, while balancing other objects, etc. Several beams can be arranged in connecting shapes such as letters, numbers, figures, etc., for enhanced spatial and interpretive stimulation.

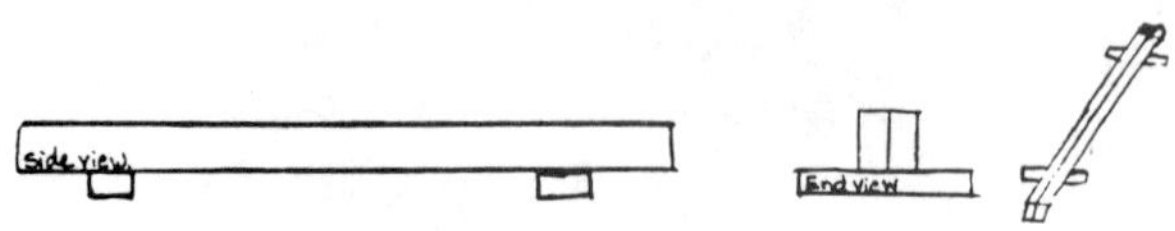


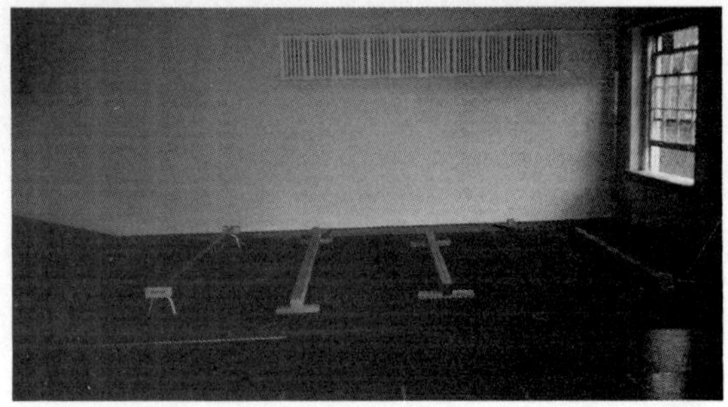

**Figure 14a–c**: Balance Beam

f. Scooter boards — If caster wheels are available, home–made scooter boards can be made easily. The more severely disabled the child, the larger the scooter board surface area should be to help provide them with enough balance and scooter surface to control their bodies. See **Figure 15**.

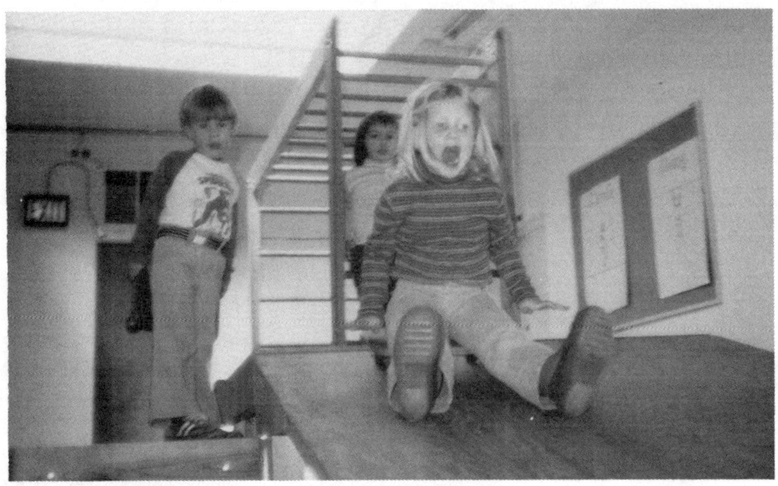

**Figure 15**: Scooter Board in use on an inclined plane

g. Slides and planes — Boards and planks can be set at inclined planes for scooter riding and climbing play (see **Figure 15).** Inclined places provide a great source of discovery with respect to which type of objects roll down easily and which do not. Inclined planes can also be carefully sanded and finished to make sliding boards.

h. See–saws — With blocks for handles and the acquisition of a stable fulcrum, a see–saw can be constructed inexpensively and easily.

i. Bowling ramps — Various sized planks and boards make effective bowling ramps for the blind or severely physically handicapped. The ramp can be used in such games as kickball, shuffleboard, and modified horseshoes, as well.

j. Adapted ping–pong — Boards can be mounted along the sides of a ping–pong table to help keep the ball in play so that the game is not interrupted so often for ball retrieval. Also, the net can be raised and the rules changed slightly to require the players to send (roll) the ball to each other under the net, instead of over it; this is another way to minimize the game's potential frustrations by players with more severe limitations.

3. HOOPS: Hoops are another very versatile type of equipment. See **Table 3** (Page 50).

a. Skip trainers — Children having difficulty learning how to skip often benefit by the use of hoops. They can be placed along the floor as shown with a specific color assigned to each foot. The child is instructed to step into the appropriate hoop, then take one hop with that same foot in the same hoop, then step into the next colored hoop with the other foot, hop, and repeat the sequence. In a short time, the child will be able to increase the tempo, thereby letting the true skipping rhythm take over (step hop; step hop; step hop; etc.). See **Figure 16**.

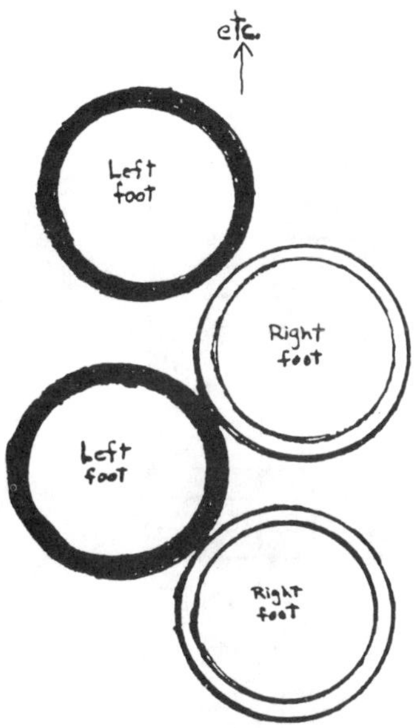


**Figure 16**: Skip Trainer

b. Target Practice — Hoops with nets attached provide for easy retrieval of projectiles. They can be placed behind other primary targets, such as pins, etc., to catch or "net" the targets and the balls, etc. Hoops standing vertically off the ground make great targets for balls, bean bags, frisbees, etc. See **Figures 17 and 18**.

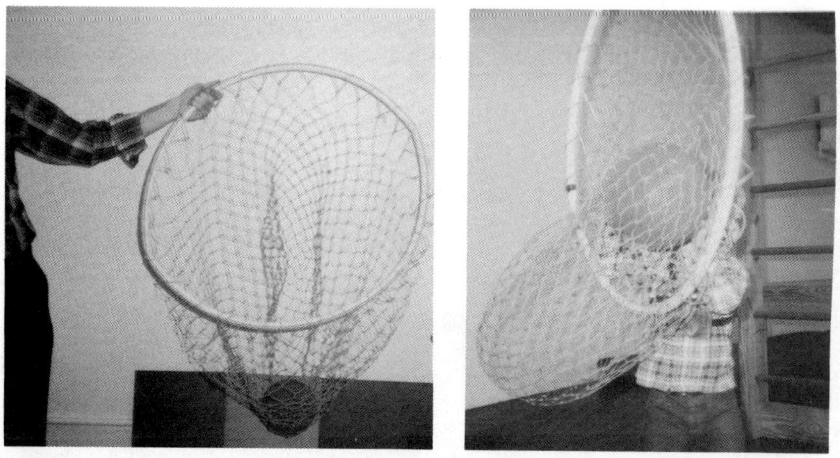

**Figure 17**: Netted Hoop Goals

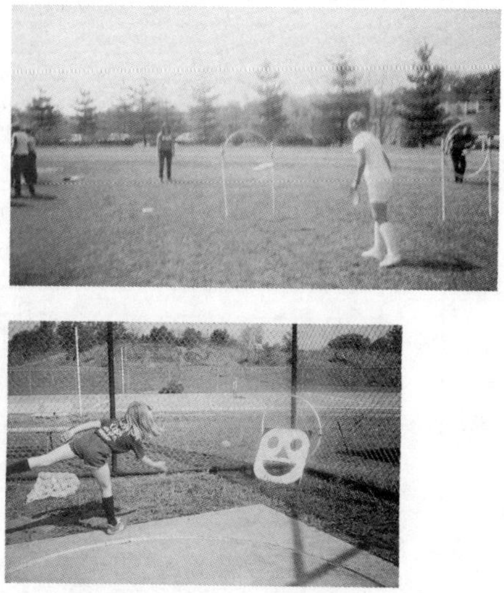

**Figure 18**: Target Hoops

Table 3: Hoops

| Hoops | Strength | Endurance | Flexibility | Relaxation | Motor Factors — | Coordination | Agility | Power | Rhythm | Developmental — | Inappropriate reflex inhibition; normal reaction facilitation | Gross Motor: locomotor skills | Gross Motor: nonlocomotor skills | Fine Motor: Prehension and manipulative skills | Sensori-Motor control |
|---|---|---|---|---|---|---|---|---|---|---|---|---|---|---|---|
| | ORGANIC | | | | NEUROMUSCULAR—PERCEPTUAL MOTOR | | | | | | | | | | |
| Skip trainers | | • | | | | • | • | | • | | • | • | • | | |
| Target practice | | | | | | • | | | | | • | | • | • | |
| Obstacles | • | • | • | | | • | • | • | • | | • | • | • | | |
| Traditional uses | • | • | • | • | | • | • | • | • | | • | • | • | • | |
| Movement exploration | • | • | • | • | | • | • | • | • | | • | • | • | • | |

| Hoops | Eye-hand/foot | Ear-hand/foot | Receipt-propulsion | Kinesthesia | Proprioception | Laterality | Directionality | Spatial Awareness | Balance — | Static | Dynamic | Vestibular | INTERPRETIVE | SOCIO-EMOTIONAL |
|---|---|---|---|---|---|---|---|---|---|---|---|---|---|---|
| | NEUROMUSCULAR—PERCEPTUAL MOTOR | | | | | | | | | | | | | |
| Skip trainers | • | • | | • | • | • | • | • | | • | • | | • | • |
| Target practice | • | | • | • | • | • | • | • | | • | • | | • | • |
| Obstacles | • | | | • | • | • | • | • | | • | • | | • | • |
| Traditional uses | • | • | • | • | • | • | • | • | | • | • | | • | • |
| Movement exploration | • | • | • | • | • | • | • | • | | • | • | • | • | • |

| Hoops | Spinal Cord Injury | Spinal Myelodysplasia | Amputations | Cerebral Palsy | Muscular Dystropy | Arthritis, arthegryposia, osteogenesis imperfecta | Temporary Conditions — | Fractures | Scoliosis, Kyphosis, Lordosis | Legg-Parthes Disease | Slipped capital Femoral Epiphysis | Diabetes | Cystic Fibrosis | Luekemia | Epilepsy | Hemophilia | Ostomies | Visually Impaired | Hearing Impaired | Developmental Delay | Clumsy Child | Educable MR | Trainable MR | Severe/profound MR | LEARNING DISABILITIES | EMOTIONALLY DISTURBED | SENIOR CITIZENS |
|---|---|---|---|---|---|---|---|---|---|---|---|---|---|---|---|---|---|---|---|---|---|---|---|---|---|---|---|
| | PHYSICAL DISABILITIES | | | | | | | | | | | MEDICAL | | | | | | SENSORY | | | | | | | | | |
| Skip trainers | — | o | o | o | o | o | o | o | + | — | — | + | o | + | + | + | + | + | + | + | + | + | + | + | + | + | + |
| Target practice | + | + | + | + | + | + | + | + | + | + | + | + | + | + | + | + | + | + | + | + | + | + | + | + | + | + | + |
| Obstacles | + | + | + | + | + | + | + | + | + | + | + | + | + | + | + | + | + | + | + | + | + | + | + | + | + | + | + |
| Traditional uses | o | o | o | o | o | o | o | o | + | o | o | + | o | + | + | + | + | + | + | + | + | + | + | + | + | + | + |
| Movement exploration | + | + | + | + | + | o | o | o | + | + | + | + | + | + | + | + | + | + | + | + | + | + | + | + | + | + | + |

c. Obstacles — Hoops can be set up alone or in long series to be used as obstacles through which to crawl, jump, dive, and swim. See **Figure 19**.

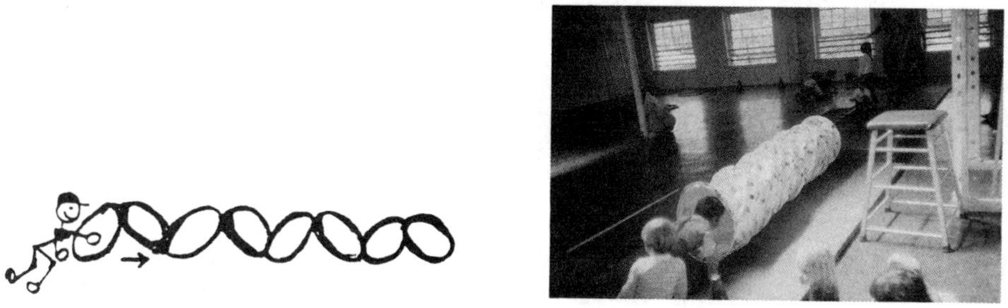

**Figure 19**: Hoop Tunnel

d. Traditional uses — Hoops can be used for hula hooping, jump roping, walking/running alongside, spin throwing to return to sender, and more. These traditional uses continue to excite the young learner.

e. Movement exploration — Hoop movement exploration, hoop dancing, hoop rhythm gymnastics, hoop relays, are just a few more examples of the many and varied activities that can be done with hoops.

4. BALLS: See **Table 4** (Page 52) for a summary of this exciting category of equipment.

a. Large therapy balls: Large rubber, vinyl or plastic balls can be used very effectively in facilitating proper balance and equilibrium reactions while positioning the body in a way to inhibit inappropriate reactions. Bright, colorful, and exciting, these balls can often provide optimal positioning and relaxation experiences for even the most severely disabled populations. See **Figure 20a–b**.

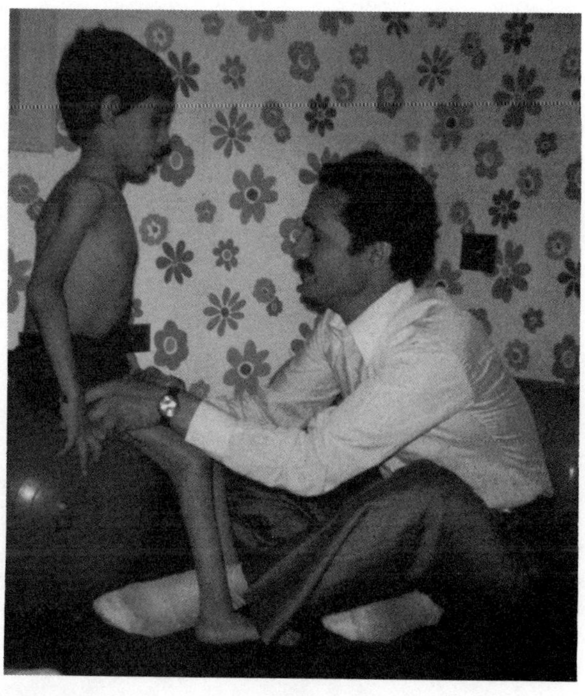

**Figure 20a**: Therapy Ball

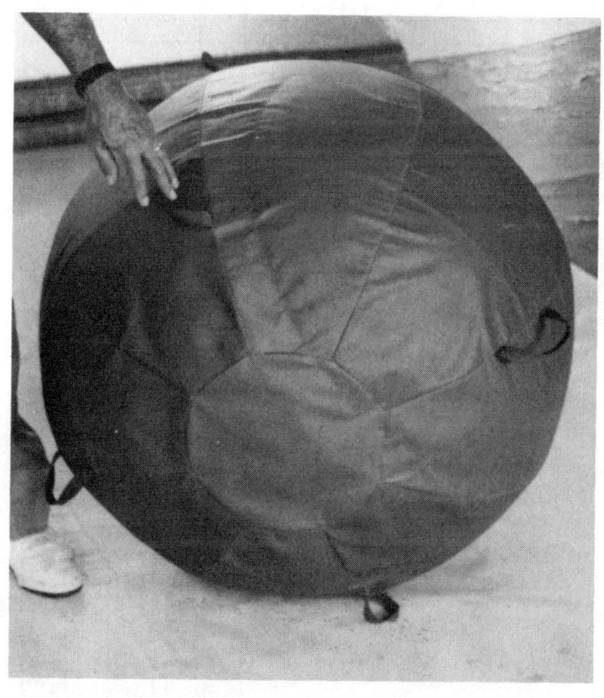

**Figure 20b**: Large Therapy Ball

| | | ORGANIC | | | | NEUROMUSCULAR—PERCEPTUAL MOTOR | | | | | | | | | | | | | | | | | | | | | | | | |
|---|---|---|---|---|---|---|---|---|---|---|---|---|---|---|---|---|---|---|---|---|---|---|---|---|---|---|---|---|---|---|
| | | Strength | Endurance | Flexibility | Relaxation | Motor Factors — | Coordination | Agility | Power | Rhythm | Developmental — | Inappropriate reflex inhibition; normal reaction facilitation | Gross Motor: locomotor skills | Gross Motor: nonlocomotor | Fine Motor: Prehension and manipulative skills | Sensori-Motor control | Eye-hand/foot | Ear-hand/foot | Receipt-propulsion | Kinesthesia | Proprioception | Laterality | Directionality | Spatial Awareness | Balance — | Static | Dynamic | Vestibular | INTERPRETIVE | SOCIO-EMOTIONAL |
| Balls | Large therapy balls | • | • | • | • | | • | • | • | • | | • | | • | | | • | | | • | • | • | • | • | | • | • | • | • | • |
| | Mdfctn organized sports/games | • | • | • | • | | • | • | • | • | | • | • | • | • | | • | • | • | • | • | • | • | • | | • | • | | • | • |
| | Implement attachment | • | • | • | • | | • | • | • | • | | • | | • | • | | • | | • | • | • | • | • | • | | • | • | | • | • |
| | Auto-rtn basketball | | • | • | • | | • | • | • | • | | • | | • | • | | • | | • | • | • | • | • | • | | • | | | • | • |
| | Tee baseball | • | • | • | • | | • | | • | | | • | | • | • | | • | | • | • | • | • | • | • | | • | | | • | • |

| | | PHYSICAL DISABILITIES | | | | | | | | | | | MEDICAL | | | | | | SENSORY | | | | | | | | | |
|---|---|---|---|---|---|---|---|---|---|---|---|---|---|---|---|---|---|---|---|---|---|---|---|---|---|---|---|---|
| | | Spinal Cord Injury | Spinal Myelodysplasia | Amputations | Cerebral Palsy | Muscular Dystropy | Arthritis, arthegryposia, osteogenesis imperfecta | Temporary Conditions — | Fractures | Scoliosis, Kyphosis, Lordosis | Legg-Parthes Disease | Slipped capital Femoral | Diabetes | Cystic Fibrosis | Luekemia | Epilepsy | Hemophilia | Ostomies | Visually Impaired | Hearing Impaired | Developmental Delay | Clumsy Child | Educable MR | Trainable MR | Severe/profound MR | LEARNING DISABILITIES | EMOTIONALLY | SENIOR CITIZENS |
| Balls | Large therapy balls | o | + | + | + | + | + | o | o | o | o | o | + | + | + | + | + | + | + | + | + | + | + | + | + | + | + | + |
| | Mdfctn organized sports/games | + | + | + | + | + | + | + | + | + | + | + | + | + | + | + | + | + | + | + | + | + | + | + | + | + | + | + |
| | Implement attachment | + | + | + | + | + | + | + | + | + | + | + | + | + | + | + | + | + | + | + | + | + | + | + | + | + | + | + |
| | Auto-rtn basketball | + | + | + | + | + | + | o | o | — | + | + | + | + | + | + | + | + | + | + | + | + | + | + | + | + | + | + |
| | Tee baseball | o | + | + | o | o | + | o | o | o | + | + | + | + | + | + | + | + | + | + | + | + | + | + | + | + | + | + |

**Table 4**: Balls

b. Modifying organized sports and games — The very young, very old, very frightened, and severely physically disabled (including quadriplegics) can enjoy and succeed in beach ball volleyball. The ball is slow, soft, safe, and easily tracked and returned even with a shrug of the shoulders, or a nod of the head even from those limited to only these motions. Balloons, tape, and newspaper balls, as well as foam (nerf) balls can also be used in modified volleyball games. In addition, badminton, kickball, soccer, baseball, and football (just to name a few) all can be modified with these softer ball ideas. See **Figure 21**.

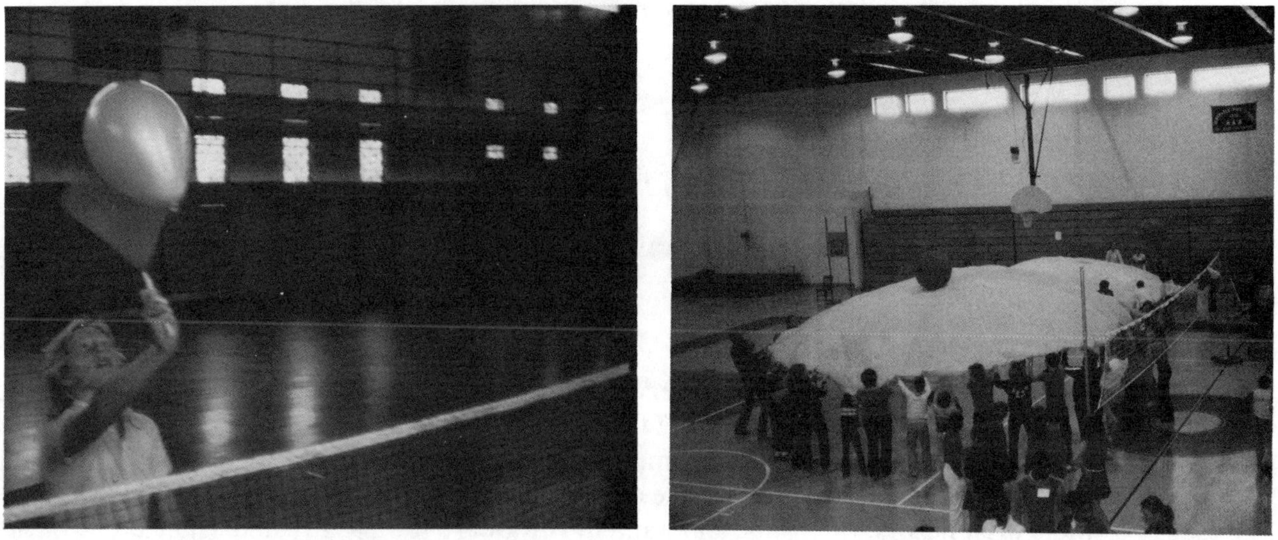

**Figure 21**: Modified Badminton

Partially deflated soccer or playground balls provide a stimulating and safe adaptation to broomball. Partially deflated footballs are easier to catch and do not feel so hard or painful by the receiver. The incorporation of larger than usual balls into wheelchair–stretcher hockey or soccer increases the frequency of successful contacts and general ball control. Regulation hockey pucks or regulation soccer balls would be rarely seen or controlled by students in electric wheelchairs, stretchers, or students who are significantly mentally and/or sensorily impaired. See **Figures 22 and 23**.

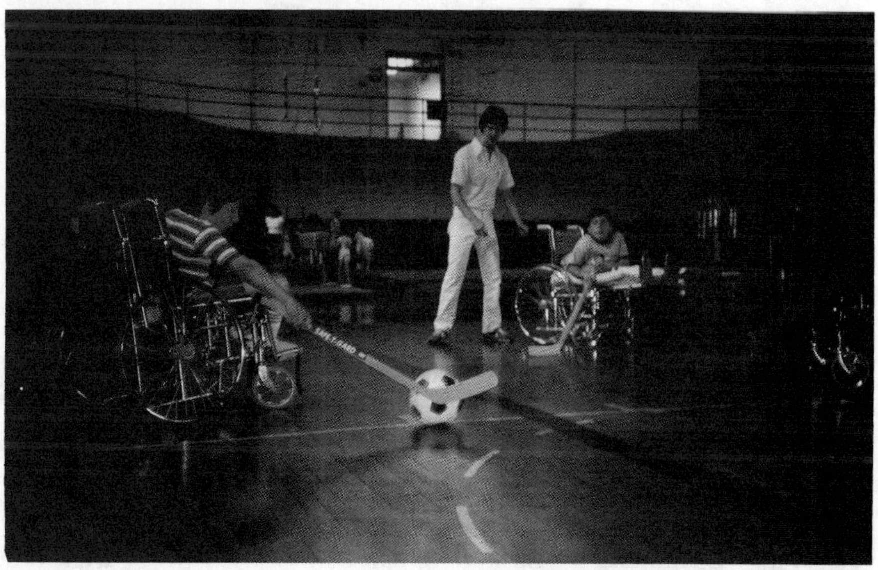

**Figure 22**: Modified Hockey

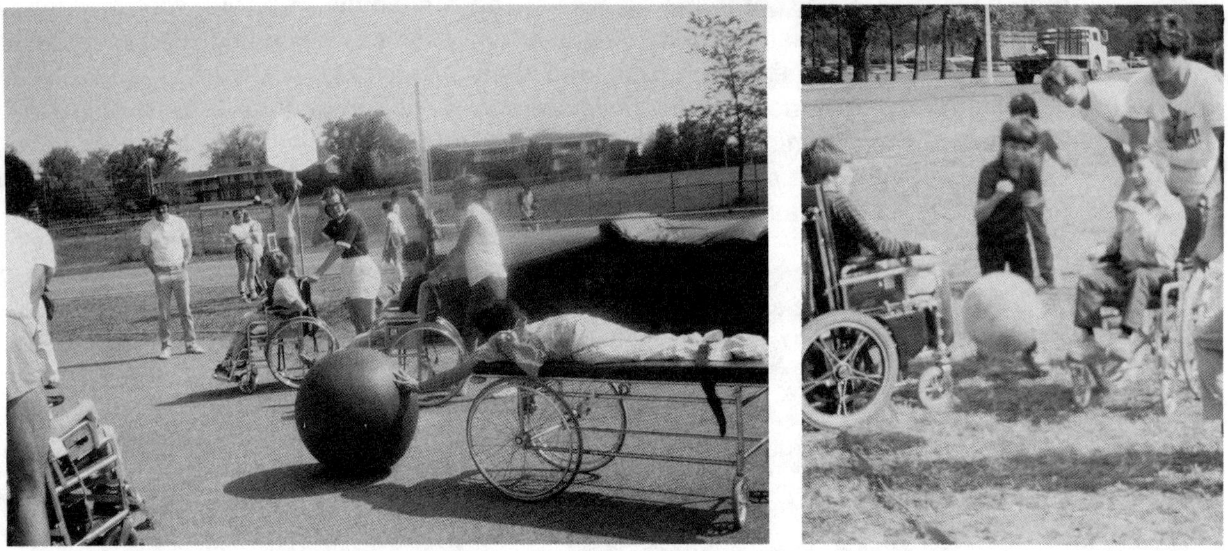

**Figure 23**: Modified Soccer

c. Fastening of implements — Racquets, paddles and bats can be fastened in a variety of simple to intricate methods. **Figure 24** shows how Velcro strips can be nailed to a paddle to accommodate most any size forearm. Individuals presenting with cerebral palsy, muscular dystrophy, or spinal cord lesions at the cervical levels (quadriplegics) can benefit in this way as their wrist flexors, extensors, and hand intrinsics are usually affected. Individuals having severe cerebral palsy, extremely advanced muscular dystrophy, or a high level of complete spinal cord lesion, however, may not have enough upper extremity function to benefit from this device (and may be limited to head, mouth, and minimal shoulder functioning, e.g., a C–4 quadriplegic, or head, mouth, and limited finger function, e.g., in advanced muscular dystrophy).

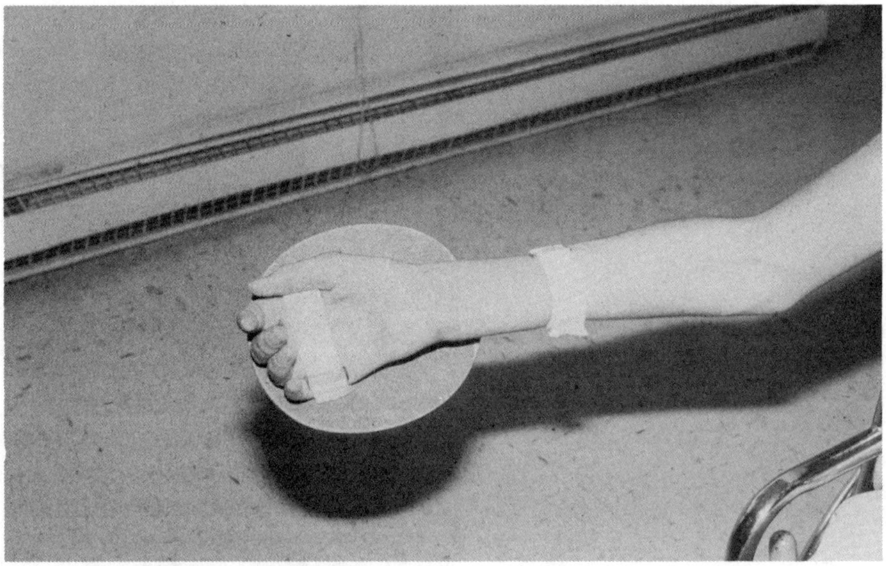

**Figure 24**: Velcro Paddle

d. Basketball — Basketball can be modified in regards to closed (independent) versus open (more than one person having an effect on the environment) organization. Ball size and weight, as well as basket height and distance, can all be manipulated. Generally, the very young, beginners, or the severely mentally or physically disabled should begin with lighter balls and closer, lower baskets. As skill and confidence improve, appropriate modifications can be made. See **Figures 25 and 26**. An automatic return basketball arrangement for stretcher or wheelchair bound individuals with limited mobility can be set up quite easily. First, place the basket against a wall at an appropriate height. Next, fasten a net, or even a sheet, below and to either side of the basket. Then stretch and incline the net or sheet downward toward the shooter, fastening it to the wheelchair arm rests. Now the ball is always returned to the sender.

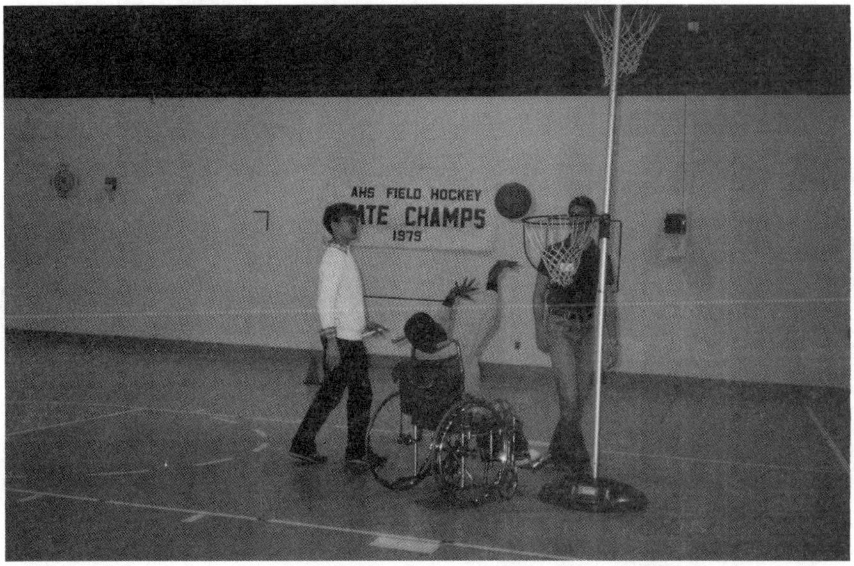


**Figure 25**: Very Low Basket Height

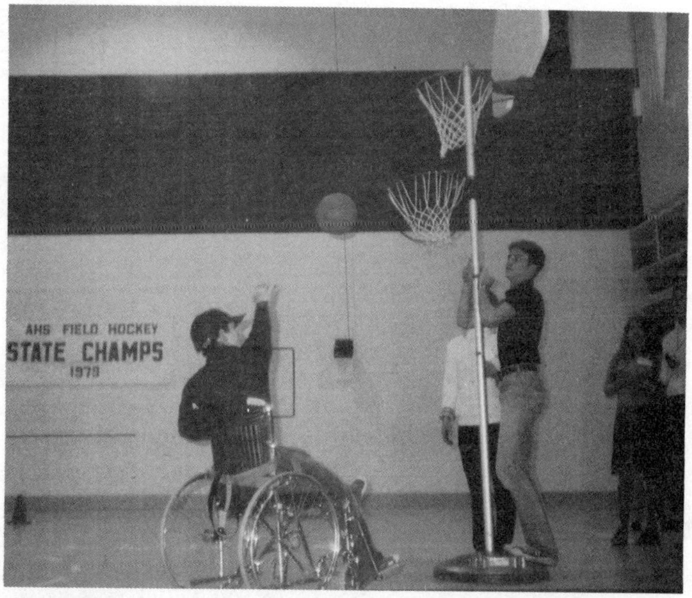


**Figure 26**: Medium Height Basketball Goal

e. <u>Tee baseball</u> — A baseball tee is a very helpful piece of equipment for both individualized and group instruction. A string can be tied to the ball for convenient retrieval. A batting tee can be easily made with a plywood base, or even an automobile wheel. A pole, dowel, or even an old plastic bat, cut at the top end to hold a ball, can be positioned to serve as the tee. Large traffic cones make excellent tees; they are inexpensive, lightweight, and stable. Generally, beginners need bigger balls as targets to hit off the tee. As their skills progress, appropriate modifications can be made with respect to decreasing the ball size (to using even regulation baseballs and softballs) and integrating them into group tee ball games. See **Figures 27 and 28**.

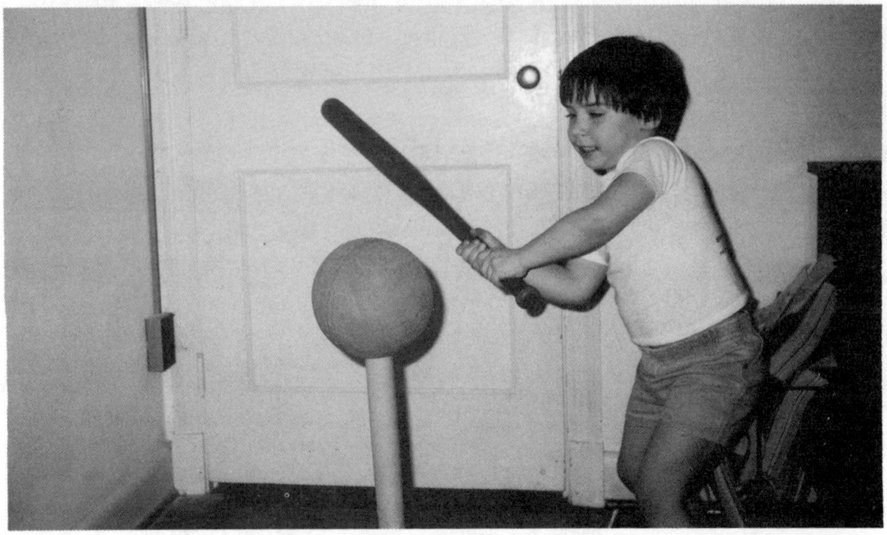

**Figure 27**: Beginning Tee Ball

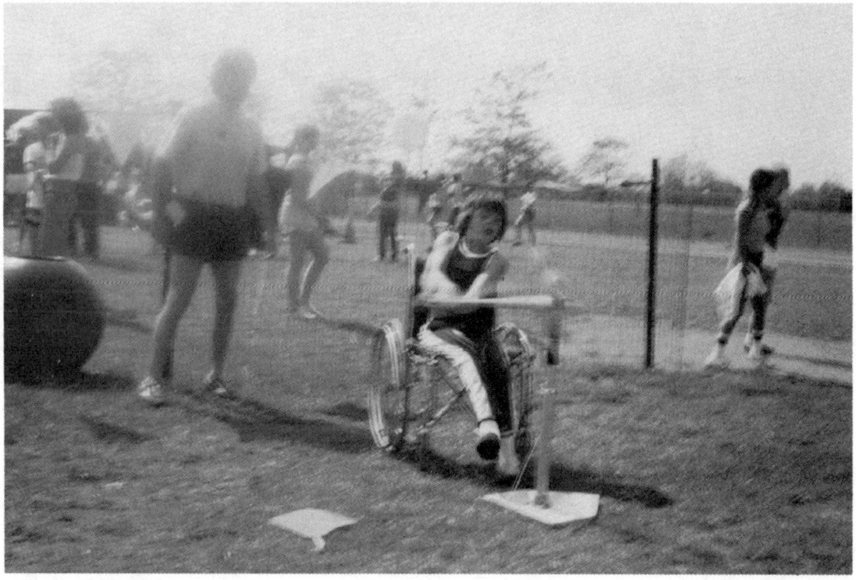

**Figure 28**: Advanced Tee Ball

If the student is especially physically limited, the batting tee itself can be adapted to incorporate a spring loaded plastic bat, set to be cocked and when released. It is set to accurately strike the ball on the tee. Depending on the desire of the participants, various sizes of springs can be used, the larger ones resulting in balls being hit faster and farther. See **Figure 29**. To construct such an adapted (automatic) batting tee, the universal flinger mechanism (discussed in Part One for the Fishing Apparatus and the Frisbee Thrower) is utilized. A plastic bat is fastened to the flinger arm which is mounted to "fling" or "swing" horizontally. A tee is attached at a height and position to result in a properly directed hit when the ball is struck by the flinger directed bat. The child only needs to be able to pull the flinger back, release it, and get ready to "run the bases" due to his/her ensuing home run.

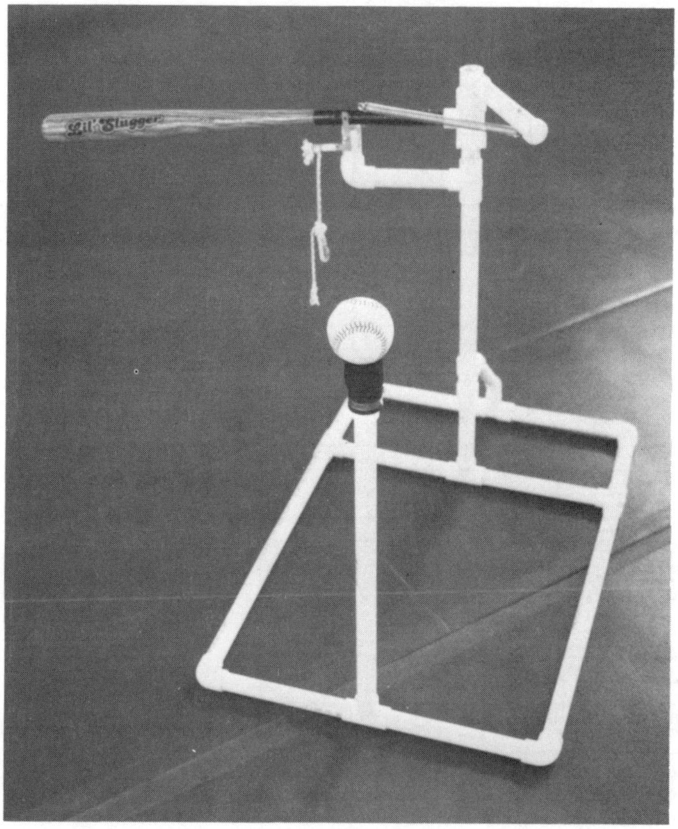


**Figure 29**: Automatic Tee Ball

5. PLASTIC BOTTLES: Plastic bottles are extremely versatile. See **Table 5** (Page 58).

   a. Scoops — Plastic bottles can be cut in a way to make very effective implements for receipt and propulsion for balls, bean bags, etc., for individual, partner, or group activities. In addition, these scoops can be used as shovels for sand, pebbles, marbles, etc.

   b. Cones — Plastic bottles can conveniently serve as obstacle course markers, goal markers, end zone markers, etc.

   c. Exercise — The bottles can be filled with varying amounts of sand and used as exercise weights.

   d. Arts and crafts — The bottles can be painted or decorated into a variety of entertaining and useful animate or inanimate objects.

   e. Target practice — Plastic bottles may be easily utilized as safe and effective targets for rolling, throwing, and kicking games (e.g., pitching practice, bowling, etc.).

   f. Floaties — A 3 foot string tied to two 2 liter bottles (gallon bottles for adults), allows for the child to lie supine, comfortably and securely, in the water with the bottles floating between the arm and chest. The air filled bottles are effective, versatile, and very inexpensive floatation devices. See **Figure 30**.

| Plastic Bottles | ORGANIC | | | | NEUROMUSCULAR—PERCEPTUAL MOTOR | | | | | | | | | | | | | | | | | | | | | | |
|---|---|---|---|---|---|---|---|---|---|---|---|---|---|---|---|---|---|---|---|---|---|---|---|---|---|---|---|
| | Strength | Endurance | Flexibility | Relaxation | Motor Factors — | Coordination | Agility | Power | Rhythm | Developmental — | Inappropriate reflex inhibition; normal reaction facilitation | Gross Motor: locomotor skills | Gross Motor: nonlocomotor skills | Fine Motor: Prehension and manipulative skills | Sensori-Motor control | Eye-hand/foot | Ear-hand/foot | Receipt-propulsion | Kinesthesia | Proprioception | Laterality | Directionality | Spatial Awareness | Balance — | Static | Dynamic | Vestibular |
| Scoops | | • | • | | | • | • | | • | | • | | • | | | • | | • | • | • | • | • | • | | • | | |
| Cones | • | • | • | • | | • | • | • | | | • | • | • | | | • | | • | • | • | • | • | • | | • | • | |
| Exerciser | • | • | • | • | | • | | • | | | • | | • | | | • | | • | • | • | • | • | • | | • | | |
| Arts and Crafts | | | | • | | • | | | • | | • | | | • | | • | • | | • | • | • | • | • | | • | | |
| Target practice | • | • | | | | • | | | | | • | | • | | | • | • | • | • | • | • | • | • | | • | | |
| Storage | | | | • | | | | | | | | | | | | | | | | | | | | | | | |

| Plastic Bottles | INTERPRETIVE | SOCIO-EMOTIONAL | PHYSICAL DISABILITIES | | | | | | | | | | |
|---|---|---|---|---|---|---|---|---|---|---|---|---|---|
| | | | Spinal Cord Injury | Spinal Myelodysplasia | Amputations | Cerebral Palsy | Muscular Dystropy | Arthritis, arthegryposia, osteogenesis imperfecta | Temporary Conditions — | Fractures | Scoliosis, Kyphosis, Lordosis | Legg-Parthes Disease | Slipped capital Femoral Epiphysis |
| Scoops | • | • | o | + | + | + | o | + | + | + | + | + | + |
| Cones | • | • | o | + | + | + | o | + | + | + | + | + | + |
| Exerciser | • | • | + | + | + | + | + | + | + | + | + | + | + |
| Arts and Crafts | • | • | + | + | + | + | + | + | + | + | + | + | + |
| Target practice | • | • | + | + | + | + | + | + | + | + | + | + | + |
| Storage | | | | | | | | | | | | | |

| Plastic Bottles | MEDICAL | | | | | | SENSORY | | | | | | | | | |
|---|---|---|---|---|---|---|---|---|---|---|---|---|---|---|---|---|
| | Diabetes | Cystic Fibrosis | Luekemia | Epilepsy | Hemophilia | Ostomies | Visually Impaired | Hearing Impaired | Developmental Delay | Clumsy Child | Educable MR | Trainable MR | Severe/profound MR | LEARNING DISABILITIES | EMOTIONALLY DISTURBED | SENIOR CITIZENS |
| Scoops | + | + | + | + | + | + | + | + | + | + | + | + | + | + | + | + |
| Cones | + | + | + | + | + | + | + | + | + | + | + | + | + | + | + | + |
| Exerciser | + | + | + | + | + | + | + | + | + | + | + | + | + | + | + | + |
| Arts and Crafts | + | + | + | + | + | + | + | + | + | + | + | + | + | + | + | + |
| Target practice | + | + | + | + | + | + | + | + | + | + | + | + | + | + | + | + |
| Storage | | | | | | | | | | | | | | | | |

**Table 5**: Plastic Bottles

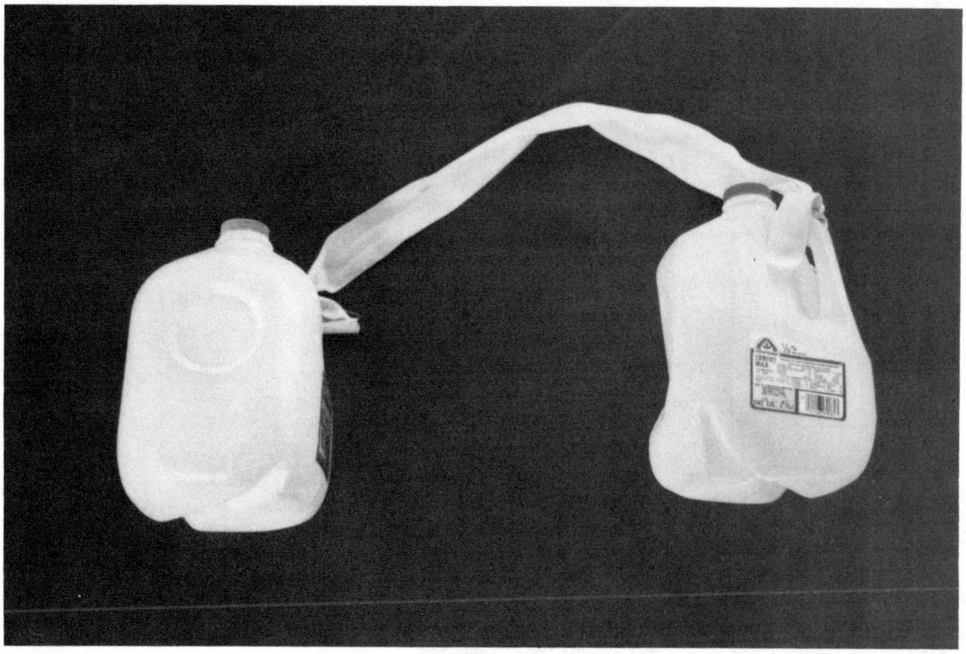

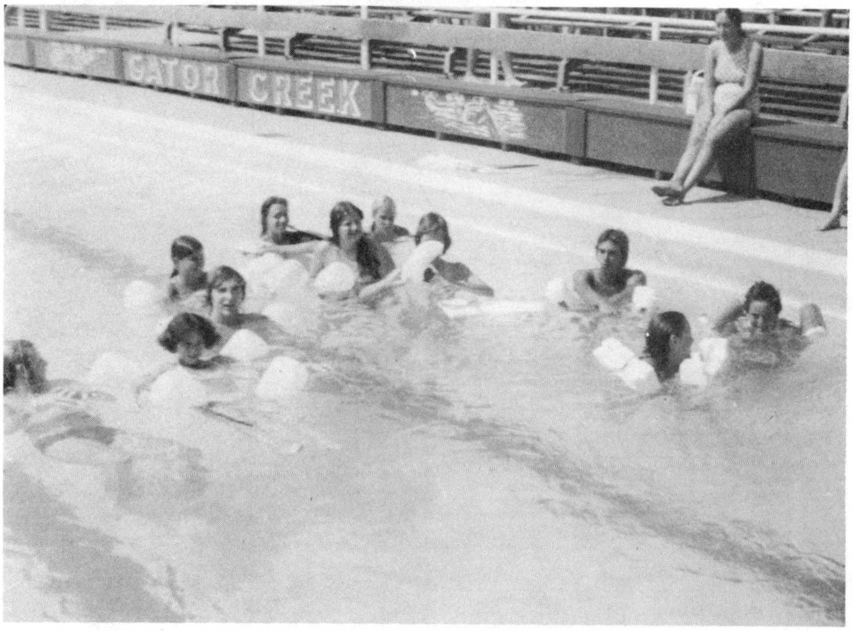


**Figure 30**: Adapted Floaties

g. Storage — When the activities are finished, the bottles — which have their tops cut off — make great storage containers as they not only hold balls, bean bags, etc., but they are self–stacking.

6. SMALL OBJECTS: Small objects such as dowels, rings, blocks, bean bags and yarn balls are very effective in facilitating the development of prehensile skills. The developmental sequence for grasping is as follows: primitive squeeze, palmer or squeeze grasp, radial–digital or inferior forefinger grasp, inferior pincer grasp, neat pincer or forefinger grasp, opposition or superior forefinger grasp. See **Table 6** (Page 60).

| Small Objects | | In general | Beanbags | Dowels | Yarnballs |
|---|---|---|---|---|---|
| ORGANIC | Strength | • | | | • |
| | Endurance | • | • | | • |
| | Flexibility | • | • | | |
| | Relaxation | • | • | | • |
| NEUROMUSCULAR—PERCEPTUAL MOTOR | Motor Factors — | | | | |
| | Coordination | • | • | • | • |
| | Agility | • | • | | |
| | Power | • | • | | |
| | Rhythm | • | • | • | |
| | Developmental — | | | | |
| | Inappropriate reflex inhibition; normal reaction facilitation | • | • | • | • |
| | Gross Motor: locomotor skills | • | • | • | • |
| | Gross Motor: nonlocomotor skills | • | • | • | • |
| | Fine Motor: Prehension and manipulative skills | • | • | • | • |
| | Sensori-Motor control | | | | |
| | Eye-hand/foot | • | • | • | • |
| | Ear-hand/foot | • | • | | |
| | Receipt-propulsion | • | • | • | • |
| | Kinesthesia | • | • | • | • |
| | Proprioception | • | • | • | • |
| | Laterality | • | • | • | • |
| | Directionality | • | • | • | • |
| | Spatial Awareness | • | • | • | • |
| | Balance — | | | | |
| | Static | • | • | • | • |
| | Dynamic | | • | • | • |
| | Vestibular | | • | • | • |
| | INTERPRETIVE | • | • | • | • |
| | SOCIO-EMOTIONAL | • | • | • | • |
| PHYSICAL DISABILITIES | Spinal Cord Injury | + | + | + | + |
| | Spinal Myelodysplasia | + | + | + | + |
| | Amputations | + | + | + | + |
| | Cerebral Palsy | + | + | + | + |
| | Muscular Dystropy | + | + | + | + |
| | Arthritis, arthegryposia, osteogenesis imperfecta | + | + | + | + |
| | Temporary Conditions — | + | + | + | + |
| | Fractures | + | + | + | + |
| | Scoliosis, Kyphosis, Lordosis | + | + | + | + |
| | Legg-Parthes Disease | + | + | + | + |
| | Slipped capital Femoral Epiphysis | + | + | + | + |
| MEDICAL | Diabetes | + | + | + | + |
| | Cystic Fibrosis | + | + | + | + |
| | Luekemia | + | + | + | + |
| | Epilepsy | + | + | + | + |
| | Hemophilia | + | + | + | + |
| | Ostomies | + | + | + | + |
| SENSORY | Visually Impaired | + | + | + | + |
| | Hearing Impaired | + | + | + | + |
| | Developmental Delay | + | + | + | + |
| | Clumsy Child | + | + | + | + |
| | Educable MR | + | + | + | + |
| | Trainable MR | + | + | + | + |
| | Severe/profound MR | + | + | + | + |
| | LEARNING DISABILITIES | + | + | + | + |
| | EMOTIONALLY DISTURBED | + | + | + | + |
| | SENIOR CITIZENS | + | + | + | + |

**Table 6**: Small Objects

a. Bean bags — Bean bags help to stimulate fine motor skills, are not intimidating objects to learn initial receipt and propulsion skills, are excellent to use as a secondary task (balancing device) in balancing skills, and can be rather effective stimulators of tactile and auditory perception.

b. Dowels — Dowels can be utilized alone as lummi sticks, rhythm sticks, perceptual motor wands for balance and gross motor skills, exercise wands, *or* in conjunction with other materials like crepe paper, ribbon or rope in the construction of Chinese ribbon dance wands (rhythmic gymnastics ribbon wands), or rope ladders, and more.

c. Yarn balls — Yarn balls make especially good lead–up substitutes for balls, badminton birdies, etc., when these skills are being introduced. They are less expensive than purchasing nerf balls.

7. RHYTHM AND MUSIC: These instruments are limited in type and number only by the imagination. See **Table 7** (Page 62).

a. Tambourines — Can be made with pebbles or dried corn inside two aluminum pie pans. Another type of tambourine can be made by stringing a stiff wire through bottle caps in a circle. A third, fancier version can be fashioned from an embroidery hoop, muslin, and bottle caps nailed around the edges.

b. Drums — Coffee cans, popcorn cans, oatmeal cartons, ice cream cartons, all provide the basic frame for building a drum. If the bottom is removed, the drum is louder.

c. Kazoos — Don't forget to hum with a comb and paper. The comb kazoo makes for a loud, convenient, simple, inexpensive and faithful horn.

8. AQUATICS: Frequently, the use of various devices and toys during swimming instruction can serve to focus the child's attention *away* from being frightened by the water and *onto* the specific toy or task at hand. Children will often bob and dive for toys when they otherwise would refuse to get their faces wet. Also, certain floatation devices serve therapeutic purposes in providing for optimal body positioning to facilitate relaxation as well as the inhibition of inappropriate patterns of movement. See **Table 8** (Page 63).

a. Floatation devices — This category includes vests, water wings, masks, goggles, snorkels, fins, lifesaving tubes, etc. These can be utilized to stimulate relaxation and improve confidence, thereby providing for the optimal conditions for learning to take place.

b. Inner tubes, rafts, and floatable toys — Floatable toys often help children overcome their fear of the water when they see that their special toy does not sink away. Furthermore, many physically disabled children have walked, hopped, jumped, and leaped for their first time ever, in pursuit of their special toy as it floats by them. The 80% reduction in the force of gravity *allows* for such achievements to take place, but the special toy is often the *catalyst* for this small miracle.

c. Sinkable toys — Objects that sink like pennies or small rocks are helpful aids in teaching children to submerge, swim to the bottom, and ascend again. Children learn that they can take control of this new environment. Toys that open and close like plastic eggs can be opened and filled with water allowing them to be either unsinkable, or sinkable, depending upon the need at hand.

d. Hoops — Hoops are great for "musical bob under your hoop" games, underwater obstacle course swims, target practice, relays races, and more.

| Music | Strength | Endurance | Flexibility | Relaxation | Motor Factors — Coordination | Agility | Power | Rhythm | Developmental | Inappropriate reflex inhibition; | Gross Motor: | Gross Motor: | Fine Motor: Prehension and | Sensori-Motor | Eye-hand/foot | Ear-hand/foot | Receipt-propulsio | Kinesthesia | Proprioception | Laterality | Directionality | Spatial | Balance — | Static | Dynamic | Vestibular |
|---|---|---|---|---|---|---|---|---|---|---|---|---|---|---|---|---|---|---|---|---|---|---|---|---|---|---|
| | ORGANIC | | | | NEUROMUSCULAR—PERCEPTUAL MOTOR | | | | | | | | | | | | | | | | | | | | | |
| Tambourines | | • | | • | • | | | • | | | | | • | | • | | | • | • | • | • | • | | | | |
| Drums | | • | • | • | • | | | • | | | | | • | | • | | | • | • | • | • | • | | | | |
| Kazoos | | | | • | • | | | • | | | | | • | | • | | | • | • | | | | | | | |

| Music | INTERPRETIVE | SOCIO-EMOTI | | Spinal Cord | Spinal | Amputations | Cerebral Palsy | Muscular | Arthritis, arthegryposia, | Temporary | Fractures | Scoliosis, | Legg-Parthes | Slipped capital |
|---|---|---|---|---|---|---|---|---|---|---|---|---|---|---|
| | | | | PHYSICAL DISABILITIES | | | | | | | | | | |
| Tambourines | • | • | | + | + | o | o | o | + | + | + | + | + | + |
| Drums | • | • | | o | + | o | o | o | + | + | + | + | + | + |
| Kazoos | • | • | | + | + | + | + | + | + | + | + | + | + | + |

| Music | Diabetes | Cystic Fibrosis | Luekemia | Epilepsy | Hemophilia | Ostomies | Visually Impaired | Hearing Impaired | Developmental | Clumsy Child | Educable MR | Trainable MR | Severe/profound | LEARNING | EMOTIONALL | SENIOR |
|---|---|---|---|---|---|---|---|---|---|---|---|---|---|---|---|---|
| | MEDICAL | | | | | | SENSORY | | | | | | | | | |
| Tambourines | + | + | + | + | + | + | + | + | + | + | + | + | + | + | + | + |
| Drums | + | + | + | + | + | + | + | + | + | + | + | + | + | + | + | + |
| Kazoos | + | + | + | + | + | + | + | + | + | + | + | + | + | + | + | + |

**Table 7**: Rhythm and Music

| Aquatics | ORGANIC | | | | NEUROMUSCULAR—PERCEPTUALMOTOR | | | | | | | | | | | | | | | | | | | | | | | | |
|---|---|---|---|---|---|---|---|---|---|---|---|---|---|---|---|---|---|---|---|---|---|---|---|---|---|---|---|---|---|
| | Strength | Endurance | Flexibility | Relaxation | Motor Factors — | Coordination | Agility | Power | Rhythm | Developmental — | Inappropriate reflex inhibition; normal reaction facilitation | Gross Motor: locomotor skills | Gross Motor: nonlocomotor skills | Fine Motor: Prehension and manipulative skills | Sensori-Motor control | Eye-hand/foot | Ear-hand/foot | Receipt-propulsion | Kinesthesia | Proprioception | Laterality | Directionality | Spatial Awareness | Balance — | Static | Dynamic | Vestibular | INTERPRETIVE | SOCIO-EMOTIONAL |
| In general | • | • | • | • | | • | • | • | • | | • | • | • | • | | • | • | • | • | • | • | • | • | | • | • | • | • | • |
| Flotation devices | | • | | • | | • | | | | | • | • | • | | | • | | • | • | • | • | • | • | | • | • | • | • | • |
| Masks and goggles | | | | • | | • | | | | | • | • | • | | | • | | | • | • | • | • | • | | • | • | • | • | • |
| Snorkels | | | | • | | • | | | | | • | • | • | • | | • | | | • | • | • | • | • | | • | • | • | • | • |
| Fins | • | • | • | • | | • | • | • | • | | • | • | | | | | | | • | • | • | • | • | | • | • | • | • | • |
| Inner tubes | • | • | • | • | | • | • | • | • | | • | • | • | | | • | | | • | • | • | • | • | | • | • | • | • | • |
| Hoops | | • | • | • | | • | • | • | • | | • | • | • | • | | • | | • | • | • | • | • | • | | • | • | • | • | • |
| Floatable toys | | • | • | • | | • | • | • | • | | • | • | • | • | | • | • | • | • | • | • | • | • | | • | • | • | • | • |
| Sinkable toys | | • | • | • | | • | • | • | • | | • | • | • | • | | • | • | • | • | • | • | • | • | | • | • | • | • | • |
| Kickboards | • | • | • | • | | • | • | • | • | | • | • | | • | | • | • | • | • | • | • | • | • | | • | • | • | • | • |
| Special tricks | • | • | • | • | | • | • | • | • | | • | • | | • | | • | • | • | • | • | • | • | • | | • | • | • | • | • |

| Aquatics | PHYSICAL DISABILITIES | | | | | | | | | | | MEDICAL | | | | | | SENSORY | | | | | | | | | |
|---|---|---|---|---|---|---|---|---|---|---|---|---|---|---|---|---|---|---|---|---|---|---|---|---|---|---|---|
| | Spinal Cord Injury | Spinal Myelodysplasia | Amputations | Cerebral Palsy | Muscular Dystropy | Arthritis, arthegryposia, osteogenesis imperfecta | Temporary Conditions — | Fractures | Scoliosis, Kyphosis, Lordosis | Legg–Parthes Disease | Slipped capital Femoral Epiphysis | Diabetes | Cystic Fibrosis | Luekemia | Epilepsy | Hemophilia | Ostomies | Visually Impaired | Hearing Impaired | Developmental Delay | Clumsy Child | Educable MR | Trainable MR | Severe/profound MR | LEARNING DISABILITIES | EMOTIONALLY DISTURBED | SENIOR CITIZENS |
| In general | + | + | + | + | + | o | o | o | + | + | + | + | + | + | + | + | + | + | + | + | + | + | + | + | + | + | + |
| Flotation devices | + | + | + | + | + | + | o | o | + | + | + | + | + | + | + | + | + | + | + | + | + | + | + | + | + | + | + |
| Masks and goggles | + | + | + | + | + | + | o | o | + | + | + | + | + | + | + | + | + | o | + | + | + | + | + | + | + | + | + |
| Snorkels | + | + | + | o | + | + | o | o | + | + | + | + | + | + | o | o | o | + | + | + | + | + | + | + | + | + | + |
| Fins | o | o | o | o | o | o | o | o | + | o | o | + | + | + | + | + | + | + | + | + | + | + | + | + | + | + | + |
| Inner tubes | o | o | + | o | o | + | o | o | o | o | o | + | + | + | + | + | + | + | + | + | + | + | + | + | + | + | + |
| Hoops | + | + | + | + | + | + | o | o | + | + | + | + | + | + | + | + | + | + | + | + | + | + | + | + | + | + | + |
| Floatable toys | + | + | + | + | + | + | o | o | + | + | + | + | + | + | + | + | + | + | + | + | + | + | + | + | + | + | + |
| Sinkable toys | o | + | + | o | o | + | o | o | + | + | + | + | + | + | + | + | + | + | + | + | + | + | + | + | + | + | + |
| Kickboards | o | + | + | o | o | o | o | o | + | + | + | + | + | + | + | + | + | + | + | + | + | + | + | + | + | + | + |
| Special tricks | + | + | + | + | + | + | + | + | + | + | + | + | + | + | + | + | + | + | + | + | + | + | + | + | + | + | + |

**Table 8**: Aquatics

e. Kickboards — Buy some styrofoam and cut it appropriately. It is inexpensive and effective. Kickboards make effective baseball bats for blind children due to their size, rigidity and weight.

f. Special tricks — When patients with "heparin locks" are able to go swimming, the donning of two surgeon's operating gloves and tape gives adequate protection and comfort to the wearer without upsetting the "heparin lock." (A "heparin lock" is often worn by patients needing frequent administration of intravenous medications as the heparin serves to preclude clotting at the local injection site, e.g., leukemia chemotherapy).

9. JUMPING SKILLS: Many types of simple equipment help to invite the development of jumping skills for fun and fitness. See **Table 9** (Page 65).

a. Elastic bands — Simple elastic bands, from sewing kits, make handy and effective Chinese jump ropes.

b. Bamboo poles — Bamboo poles provide for great sticks for high jumping limbo games, and tininkling.

c. Old mattresses — Old mattresses can be utilized as mats, crash pads, and bouncing pads, where better is unavailable. Please make certain the mattresses are suitably cleaned before their use is approved.

d. Jump boards — A large plywood board affixed atop large inner tubes creates an excellent jumping board for many children at one time.

e. Jump pits — When available, the neighborhood high school or college's high jump or pole vault's crash mats provide for endless hours of jumping fun. (Please obtain permission first, and supervise the jumping closely).

f. Trampolines — If a real trampoline is available, insist on its safe utilization. In addition to its customary activities, if various colored and numbered balloons are affixed over the trampoline bed, this piece of equipment can become a sophisticated perceptual motor and academic laboratory. See **Figure 31**.

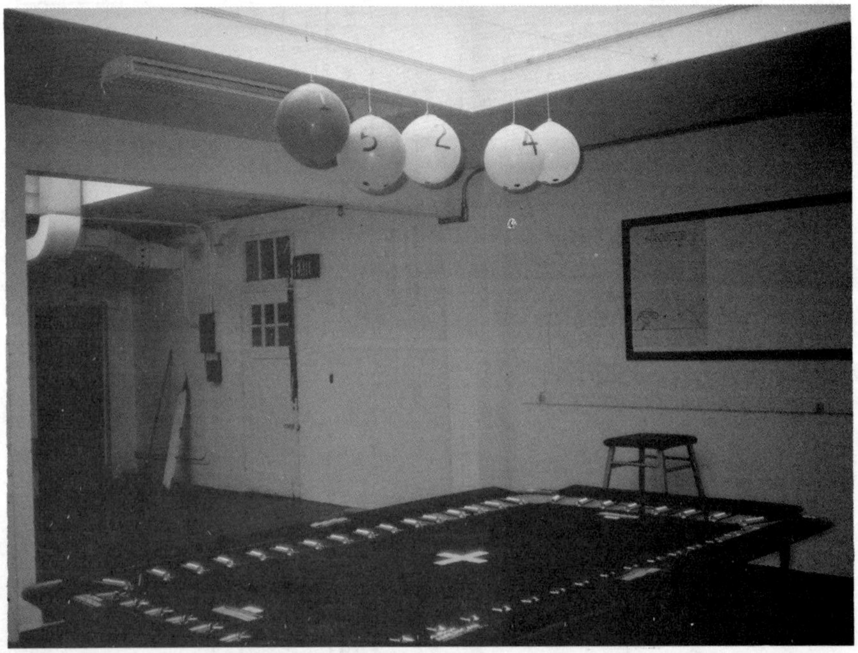

**Figure 31**: Perceptual/Psycho–Motor Trampolining

| Jumping | ORGANIC | | | | NEUROMUSCULAR—PERCEPTUALMOTOR | | | | | | | | | | | | | | | | | | | | | | |
|---|---|---|---|---|---|---|---|---|---|---|---|---|---|---|---|---|---|---|---|---|---|---|---|---|---|---|---|
| | Strength | Endurance | Flexibility | Relaxation | Motor Factors — | Coordination | Agility | Power | Rhythm | Developmental — | Inappropriate reflex inhibition; normal reaction facilitation | Gross Motor: locomotor skills | Gross Motor: nonlocomotor skills | Fine Motor: Prehension and manipulative skills | Sensori-Motor control | Eye-hand/foot | Ear-hand/foot | Receipt-propulsion | Kinesthesia | Proprioception | Laterality | Directionality | Spatial Awareness | Balance — | Static | Dynamic | Vestibular |
| Elastic bands | • | • | • | • | | • | • | • | • | | • | • | • | | | • | | | • | • | • | • | • | | • | • | • |
| Bamboo sticks | • | • | | • | | • | • | • | • | | • | • | • | • | | • | • | | • | • | • | • | • | | • | • | • |
| Mattresses | • | • | | • | | • | • | • | • | | • | • | • | | | | | | • | • | • | • | • | | • | • | • |
| Large inner tubes | • | • | | • | | • | • | • | • | | • | • | • | | | • | | | • | • | • | • | • | | • | • | • |
| High jump pits | • | • | • | • | | • | • | • | • | | • | • | | | | | | | • | • | • | • | • | | • | • | • |
| Trampolines | • | • | • | • | | • | • | • | • | | • | • | • | | | • | | | • | • | • | • | • | | • | • | • |

| Jumping | | | | PHYSICAL DISABILITIES | | | | | | | | | | | MEDICAL | | | | | |
|---|---|---|---|---|---|---|---|---|---|---|---|---|---|---|---|---|---|---|---|---|
| | INTERPRETIVE | SOCIO-EMOTIONAL | | Spinal Cord Injury | Spinal Myelodysplasia | Amputations | Cerebral Palsy | Muscular Dystropy | Arthritis, arthegryposia, osteogenesis imperfecta | Temporary Conditions — | Fractures | Scoliosis, Kyphosis, Lordosis | Legg-Parthes Disease | Slipped capital Femoral Epiphysis | Diabetes | Cystic Fibrosis | Luekemia | Epilepsy | Hemophilia | Ostomies |
| Elastic bands | • | • | | o | o | o | o | o | o | o | o | o | o | o | + | + | + | o | o | + |
| Bamboo sticks | • | • | | o | o | o | o | o | o | o | o | o | o | o | + | + | + | o | o | + |
| Mattresses | • | • | | o | o | o | o | o | o | o | o | o | o | o | + | + | + | o | o | + |
| Large inner tubes | • | • | | o | o | o | o | o | o | o | o | o | o | o | + | + | + | o | o | o |
| High jump pits | • | • | | o | o | o | o | o | o | o | o | o | o | o | + | + | + | o | o | + |
| Trampolines | • | • | | o | o | o | o | o | o | o | o | o | o | o | + | + | + | o | o | + |

| Jumping | SENSORY | | | | | | | | | |
|---|---|---|---|---|---|---|---|---|---|---|
| | Visually Impaired | Hearing Impaired | Developmental Delay | Clumsy Child | Educable MR | Trainable MR | Severe/profound MR | LEARNING DISABILITIES | EMOTIONALLY DISTURBED | SENIOR CITIZENS |
| Elastic bands | + | + | + | + | + | + | + | + | + | + |
| Bamboo sticks | + | + | + | + | + | + | + | + | + | + |
| Mattresses | + | + | + | + | + | + | + | + | + | + |
| Large inner tubes | + | + | + | + | + | + | + | + | + | + |
| High jump pits | + | + | + | + | + | + | + | + | + | + |
| Trampolines | + | + | + | + | + | + | + | + | + | + |

**Table 9**: Jumping Skills

## Summary

When working with any groups, especially special populations, the instructor should not hesitate to manipulate the environment appropriately to achieve positive and meaningful experiences. The teacher should feel free to use larger, lighter, more slow moving balls, lower baskets, increase target sizes and decrease target distances, etc., whenever indicated. At the same time, the instructor should not automatically adapt something merely because the student is disabled. Adaptations should only be used when needed and as long as they're needed. Participation without adaptations, as feasible, should be a long term goal.

Adapted equipment can be used to stimulate and facilitate new areas of learning and success. The effectiveness of the equipment is dependent upon its appropriate incorporation with respect to the specific population involved, the indicated program objectives, and the imagination and creativity of the individuals selecting and using it.

**Figure 32**, on the next pages, is a listing of the "National Handicapped Sports Chapters and Affiliates." These organizations will welcome questions from interested individuals and will provide further information to help improve programs for the disabled everywhere. In addition, the authors of this manual welcome any questions and shall try to assist in any way possible. The authors hope that the implementation of these ideas will be a truly rewarding, stimulating, and enjoyable experience for all. Good luck and have fun!

# NATIONAL HANDICAPPED SPORTS CHAPTERS AND AFFILIATES

**ALASKA**
Challenge Alaska
ATTN: Patrick Reinhart
P.O. Box 110065
Anchorage, AK 99511-0065
(907) 563-2658

Access Alaska
ATTN: Rick Tessadore
3550 Airport Way, Suite 3
Fairbanks, AK 99709
(907) 479-7940

**CALIFORNIA**
NHSRA of Southern California
The Unrecables
ATTN: Linda Fryback
2210 Glick Court
Redondo Beach, CA 90278
(213) 374-6775

San Diego Adventurers
ATTN: Kent Bry
1105 First Street
Encinitas, CA 92024
(619) 942-2188

NHSRA of Orange County
ATTN: Bob & Janet Beutner
531 Heather Avenue
La Habra, CA 90631
(231) 697-0351

NHSRA, Northern Califoria Chapter
ATTN: Douglas J. Pringle
5926 Illinois Avenue
Orangevale, CA 95662
(913) 989-0402

Cal STAR
Department of Recreational Sports
University of California
ATTN: Ann Fitzgerald
2301 Bancroft Way
Berkeley, CA 94720
(415) 642-8342

NHSRA of Fresno
ATTN: Virginia Gryalva
P.O. Box 15263
Fresno, CA 93702
(209) 252-6126

Mother Lode Chapter
ATTN: Richard K. Van Aken
P.O. Box 4274
Camp Connell, CA 95223
(209) 795-5288

**CONNECTICUT**
Connecticut Handicapped Ski Foundation
ATTN: Sal Ucello
599 Graham Road
South Windsor, CT 06074
(203) 644-1322

**COLORADO**
Breckenridge Outdoor Education Center for the Handicapped
P.O. Box 697
Breckenridge, CO 80424
(303) 453-6422

Crested Butte Physically Challenged Skier Program
ATTN: Robin Norton
P.O. Box A
Mount Crested Butte, CO 81225
(303) 349-2333

Durango/Purgatory Handicapped Sports Association
ATTN: Lisa Margol
P.O. Box 8333
Durango, CO 81301
(303) 247-9000

Rocky Mountain Handicapped Sportsmen's Assoc.
ATTN: Tom Reetz
1315 S. Eaton Ct.
Lakewood, CO 80226
(303) 934-9540

Winter Park Sports and Learning Center
ATTN: Paul Di Bello
P.O. Box 36
Winter Park, CO 80482
(303) 892-0961

Aspen Handicapped Skiers Association
ATTN: Edward H. Lucks
0174 Meadows Road
P.O. Box 5429
Snowmass Village, CO 81615
(303) 923-3294

Colorado Discovery Ability
ATTN: April Black
P.O. Box 400
Mesa, CO 81643
(303) 268-5573

Challenge West
ATTN: Rick L. Maez
1101 E. Columbia
Colorado Springs, CO 80903
(719) 630-8329

**D.C., MARYLAND, VIRGINIA**
Nation's Capitol Chapter
ATTN: Frank Stowell/Kathy Harbert
4937 West Chalk Point Road
West River, MD 20778
(301) 571-0217/868-9280/261-5075

Woodrow Wilson Rehabilitation Center
ATTN: Diane Huss
Fisherville, VA 22939
(703) 332-7000

**FLORIDA**
NHSRA, South Florida Chapter
ATTN: George DePontis
P.O. Box 370788
Miami, FL 33137
(305) 751-2525

**GEORGIA**
NHSRA, Atlanta Chapter
ATTN: Sean Shipley
P.O. Box 327
Clarkston, GA 30021
(404) 498-7204

**IDAHO**
Association for Handicapped Recreation Inc.
ATTN: Executive Director
P.O. Box 2541
Coeur d'Alene, ID 83814

Recreation Unlimited, Inc.
ATTN: Caroline Vogel
P.O. Box 447
Boise, ID 83702
(208) 383-6595

**ILLINOIS**
Chicagoland Handicapped Skiers
ATTN: Valerie Byrne
1086 Braircliffe
Wheaton, IL 60187
(312) 682-4018

**INDIANA**
Greater Indianapolis Chapter Handicapped Skiing
ATTN: Toni Williams
% Indianpolis Parks & Recreation Department
1426 West 29th Street
Indianapolis, IN 42608
(317) 634-0988

Calumet Region Chapter
ATTN: Jackson Ivery II
5032 Kennedy Avenue
East Chicago, IN 46312
(219) 391-0900

Special Outdoor Leisure Opportunities, Inc.
ATTN: Marilyn Cahalan
P.O. Box 6221
South Bend, IN 46660

**IOWA**
Sundown Handicapped Skiers
ATTN: Thomas W. Gavin
Sundown Ski Area
9000 Asbury Road
Dubuque, IA 52001
(319) 556-6676

**MASSACHUSETTS, NEW HAMPSHIRE, MAINE**
Northeast Passage Outing Club
ATTN: Jill Gravink
Northeast Rehabilitation Hospital
70 Butler Street
Salem, NH 03079
(603) 893-2900 ext, 472

Wachusett Mountain Education Foundation
ATTN: Kathy Chandler
499 Mountain Road
Princeton, MA 01541
(617) 464-5101

New England Handicapped Sportsmen's Association
ATTN: Earl Plummer
26 McFarlin Road
Chelmsford, MA 01824
(508) 256-3240

**MICHIGAN**
Michigan Handicapped Sports and Recreation Association
ATTN: Lee Helms
238 Woodview Court, Apt. 244
Rochester Hills, MI 48063-6041
(313) 853-0648

Cannonsburg Challenged Skier Association
ATTN: Theresa Rettig
1722 Widdicomb, N.W.
Grand Rapids, MI 49504
(616) 938-2391

**Figure 32**: National Handicapped Sport Chapters and Affiliates

**MINNESOTA**
Courage Alpine Skiers
ATTN: Neal Manecke
3523 Arbor Lane
Minnetonka, MN 55343
(612) 938–1724

Twin Ports Flyers
ATTN: Mary Lou Donovan
Courage Center
205 W. 2nd St., #451
Duluth, MN 55802
(218) 727–6874

**MONTANA**
I Am Third Foundation dba Eagle Mount
ATTN: Kathy Wells
P.O. Box 3118
Bozeman, MT 59772
(406) 586–1781

Dream — Big Mountain Disabled Ski Program
ATTN: Dennis Jones
P.O. Box 1058
Kalispell. MT 59903
(406) 862–3511

**NEVADA**
Northern Nevada Ski School for the Disabled
ATTN: Rosemary Dixon
P.O. Box 6244
Incline Village, NV 89450
(702) 648–2377

Lakeside Chapter, City of Las Vegas
ATTN: Roy Post
749 Veterans Memorial Drive
Las Vegas, NV 89101
(702) 648–2377

**NEW MEXICO**
Lovelace/Sandia Peak Ski Program
ATTN: Pat McGowan
2425 Ridgecrest Drive SE
Albuquerque, NM 87108
(505) 766–4755

**NEW YORK**
NHSRA of New York
ATTN: Dick Weirman
508 Verna Drive
Endwell, NY 13760
(607) 758–6960

Disabled Ski Program at Ski Windham
ATTN: Gwen C.B. Allard
EPSIA Educational Foundation
1–A Lincoln Avenue
Albany, NY 12205–4900
(518) 452–6095

**NORTH CAROLINA**
YMCA Wake County, Inc.
ATTN: Candice Matthews
1012 Oberlin Road
Raleigh NC 27065
(919) 828–3205

**OHIO**
Three Trackers of Ohio
ATTN: Joan Seitz
562 Elko Avenue
Akron, OH 44305
(216) 733–1525

**OREGON**
Flying Outriggers Ski Club
ATTN: Jolene M. Corey
211 Oregon Pioneer Building
Portland, OR 97204–2672
(503) 222–1327

Mount Hood Handicap Ski Association, Inc.
ATTN: Ralph Summers
P.O. Box 15071
Portland, OR 97217
(503) 230–6108

Shared Outdoor Adventure Recreation
P.O. Box 14583
ATTN: Dave Espeseth
Portland, OR 98214
(503) 283–1613

**PENNSYLVANIA**
Three Rivers Adaptive Sports
% Harmersville Rehabilitation Center
ATTN: Harry Skaggs
P.O. Box 11460, Guys Run Road
Pittsburgh, PA 15238
(412) 535–1389

The Philadelphia Area Handicapped Skiing Club
ATTN: Isobel Bohn/Ned Goodrich
P.O. Box 884, 28 Simpson Road
Ardmore, PA 19003
(215) 848–3666

Good Shepherd Rehabilitation Hospital
ATTN: Sarah Boyer, CTRA
T.R. Department
5th and St. John Streets
Allentown, PA 18103

Deutsch Institute Applied Research Center
ATTN: Deborah Moran
403 Chamber of Commerce Building
Mulberry and Washington Avenue
Scranton, PA 18503
(717) 348–1968

**SOUTH CAROLINA**
Palmetto Players
ATTN: Linda Lake
212 Netherland Drive
Irmo, SC 29063
(803) 781–6834

**TEXAS**
Southwest Wheelchair Athletic Association
ATTN: Judy Einbinder
1475 West Gray, Suite 161
Houston, TX 77019
(713) 522–9769

**UTAH**
Paul Hill Adaptive Sports Association
ATTN: Quintin Gray
98 Roosevelt Avenue
American Forks, UT 84003
(801) 756–5537

Park City Handicapped Sports Association
ATTN: Meeche White
P.O. Box 680286
Park City, UT 84068
(801) 649–3991

Utah Handicapped Skiers Association
ATTN: Steve Peterson
P.O. Box 108
Roy, UT 84067
(801) 777–4515

**VERMONT**
Vermont Handicapped Ski Foundation
ATTN: Laura C. Perry
P.O. Box 261, Rt. 44
Brownsville, VT 05037
(802) 484–7711 ext. 3005

**WASHINGTON**
Seattle Handicapped Sports & Recreation Association
ATTN: Sheri Baylin
P.O. Box 75614
Seattle, WA 98125
(206) 363–6510

**WEST VIRGINIA**
The Challenge Athletes of Silver Creek, West Virginia
ATTN: Gary Morriston
P.O. Box 150
Slatyfork, WV 26291
(304) 572–4000

# Notes

## Notes

# Notes

# Notes

# Notes

# Notes